Finger up the Bum

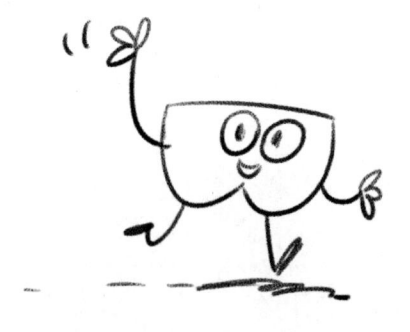

Michael Hart Izen

ILLUSTRATIONS BY **Jon Izen**
WITH **J. Roy "Sneeze" Izen**

FINGER UP THE BUM

(leola productions

Copyright © 2016 by Michael Hart Izen

Illustrations copyright © 2016 by Jon Izen and J. Roy Izen

All rights reserved. No part of this book may be reproduced, stored in a retrieval system or transmitted, in any form or by any means, without the prior written consent of the publisher or a license from The Canadian Copyright Licensing Agency (Access Copyright). For a copyright license, visit www.accesscopyright.ca or call toll free to 1-800-893-5777.

Leola Productions
Vancouver, Canada
www.ginaleolawoolsey.com

Cataloguing in Publication Data available from Library and Archives Canada

ISBN 978-0-9952787-0-7 (paperback)
ISBN 978-0-9952787-1-4 (ebook)

Cover and test design by Peter Cocking
Cover illustration by Jon Izen

16 17 18 19 20   5 4 3 2 1

This book is mostly dedicated to my darling wife, Gina.

But I can't forget the team at the Vancouver Prostate Centre and the B.C. Cancer Agency keeping me alive. Go, team, go!

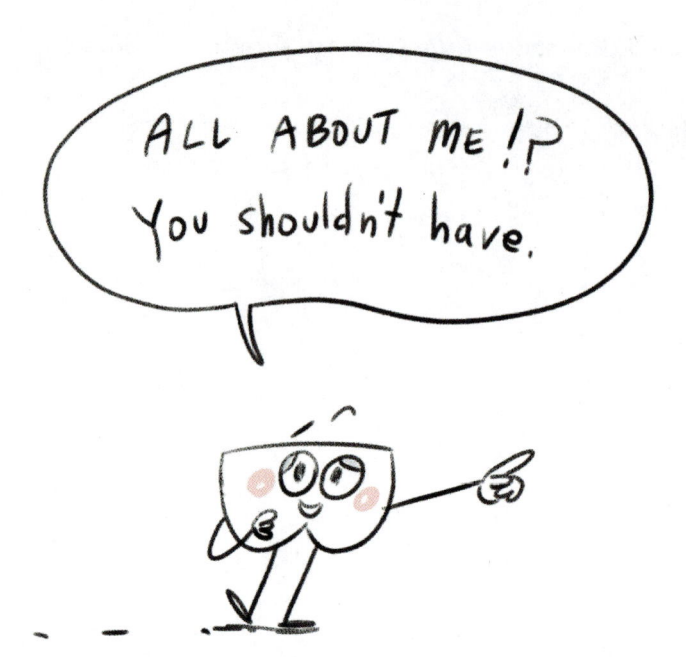

Contents

   Acknowledgments *9*

1. **Back Story: The Real Poop** *15*
2. **Problem: Softwood Lumber Issues** *19*
3. **Tests: You're Putting That Where?!?!** *25*
4. **Diagnosis: Wait, What?** *31*
5. **Surgery: I'm Still Using That** *37*
6. **Post-Surgery: What's That Coming out of My?????** *43*
7. **Hormones: Chemical Castration— That Doesn't Sound Good** *49*
8. **Radiation: The Origins of a Superhero!** *55*
9. **It's Still Not Working: Trials and Tribulations** *61*
10. **Hang on, I'm Not Dead Yet: The Meaning of Life, and Other Great Movies** *67*

   Rear End Notes: A Family Affair *71*

   Finger Fighters *74*

   Wall of Fame *77*

   About the Creators *79*

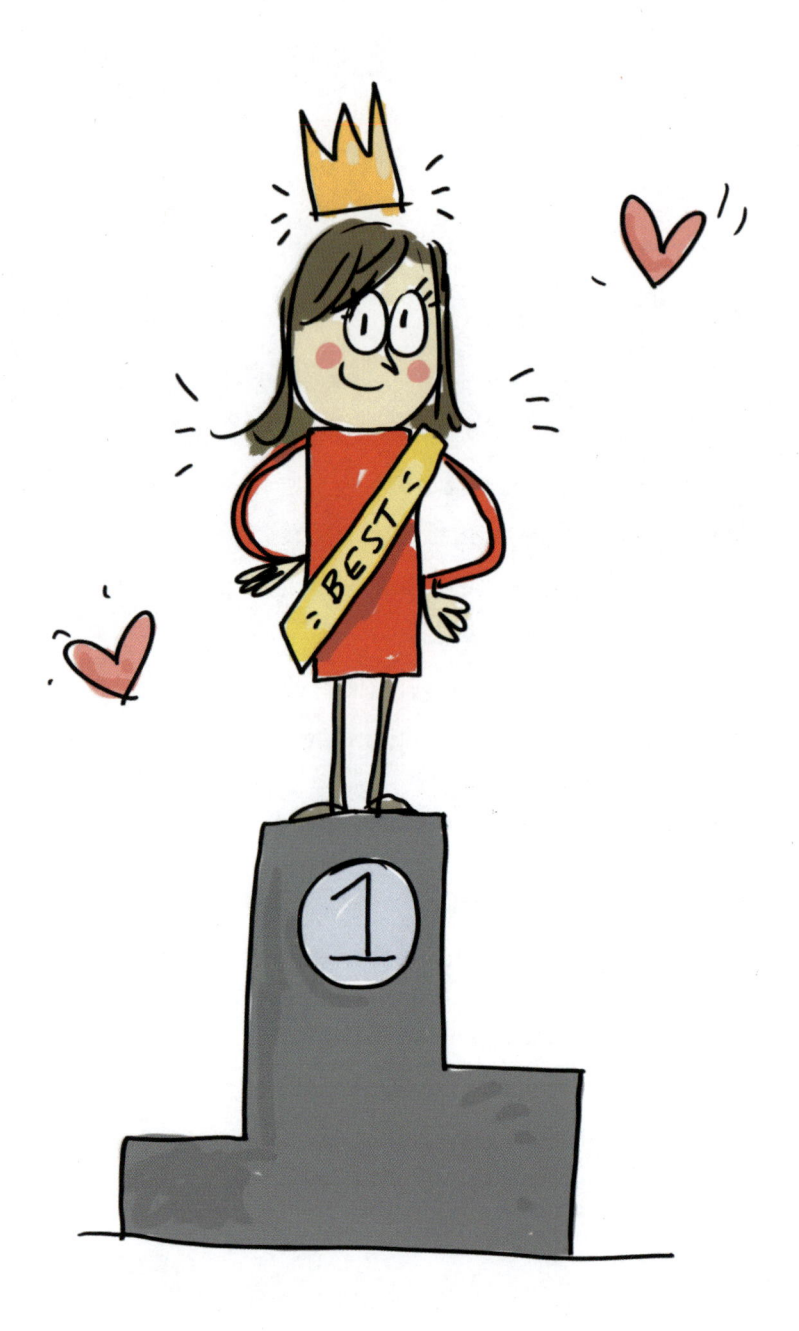

Acknowledgments

This book would not be possible without my amazing wife, Gina Leola Woolsey.

In part because she has all the writing (and most of the other) smarts in the family, and was able to take my ragtag ramblings and direct them into the almost Shakespearean tale you have in front of you right now. And in part because she did the research to recommend Page Two Strategies, Kickstarter, and other key people on this project. But mostly because she saved my life.

When I was having my initial troubles, it was Gina who kept sending me back to the doctors to get answers. When I was not always completely forthright with my doctors, it was Gina who made me tell them everything. When my doctors were content to just pass things off as one of those things, it was Gina who made us all reconsider our next course of action. When I came home from the hospital after surgery, it was Gina who nursed me back to health with good food and great care. She even got down on her hands and knees in the shower to clean the dried blood off the catheter so I wouldn't get an infection.

While I am sure your spouse is wonderful, I know mine is over-the-top incredible.

So, thank you, darling. I love you just doesn't quite cover it.

I also want to thank my brother Jon for his drawings, inspiration, and friendship... and for eventually cutting out the waterworks. It's great to have a creative partner who not only illustrates my words but also comes up with a different, yet complementary, set of ideas. You made this project a lot of fun, which is really the whole point, isn't it?

Of course my dad needs a pat on the back for his drawings, but really for setting us up as kids to appreciate both art and humor. It's a great combo. Thanks, Pops.

Hi Mom, love you, too. Thanks for putting up with three idiot sons and one infant husband. Yeah, artsy and funny is an excellent combo, unless you have to live with it.

For our crowd-funding campaign, my daughter, Chloe Woolsey, was our award-deserving director on the video, and one of the Movember Moustache Dancers. Mrs. Monica Malcolm saved my *tuchus* with her mad editing skills. The Big Z, Brad Zubyk, helped with media and led the charge for crowd-funding pledges.

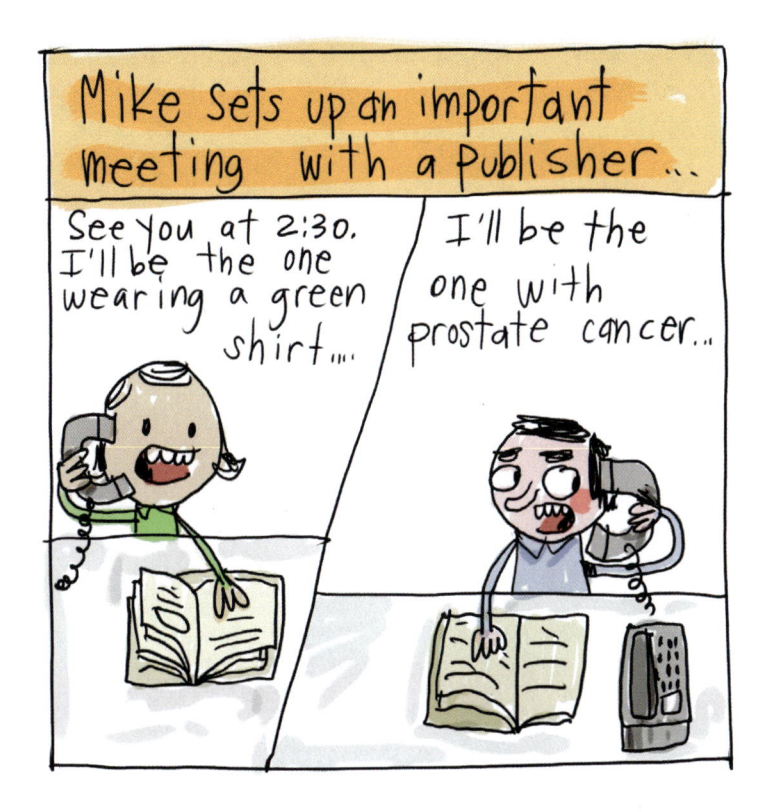

> **Mike sets up an important meeting with a publisher...**
>
> "See you at 2:30. I'll be the one wearing a green shirt...."
>
> "I'll be the one with prostate cancer..."

My personal designer, Robyn Huth, provided great graphics. (Everyone should have a personal designer.) Hometown friends Debbie Young and Gilbert Gregory really came through with media back in the 'Peg, and the incomparable Gery Lemon shared her secret stash of local contacts. Jordan Watters needs a fist-bump for helping me keep the lights on at the shop, and for the game-winning pledge. And Cousin Larry twisted every arm of close and distant relatives; he's who you want in your corner for any fundraising event.

The crowd funding itself also hooked us up with more than 250 backers, 250 supporters, 250 friends. Every pledge felt like love. Thanks.

The team at Page Two Strategies also deserves a shout-out. Thank you, Trena White, for your advice and your crack team: Shirarose Wilensky and Erin Parker for their great edits and ideas; Peter Cocking for the design, layout, and shared vision with Jon; and our fan-fave, Gabrielle Narsted, for keeping us all on the same page, too.

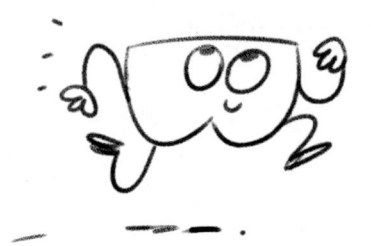

FINGER UP THE BUM

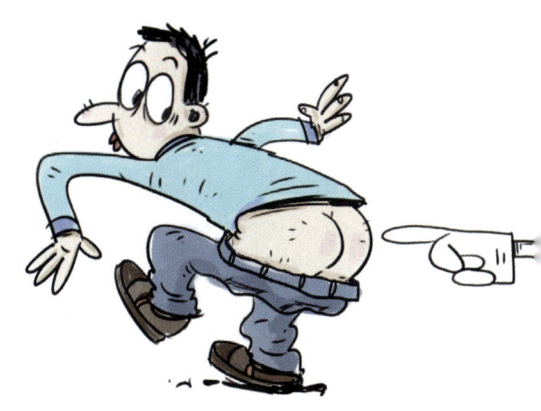

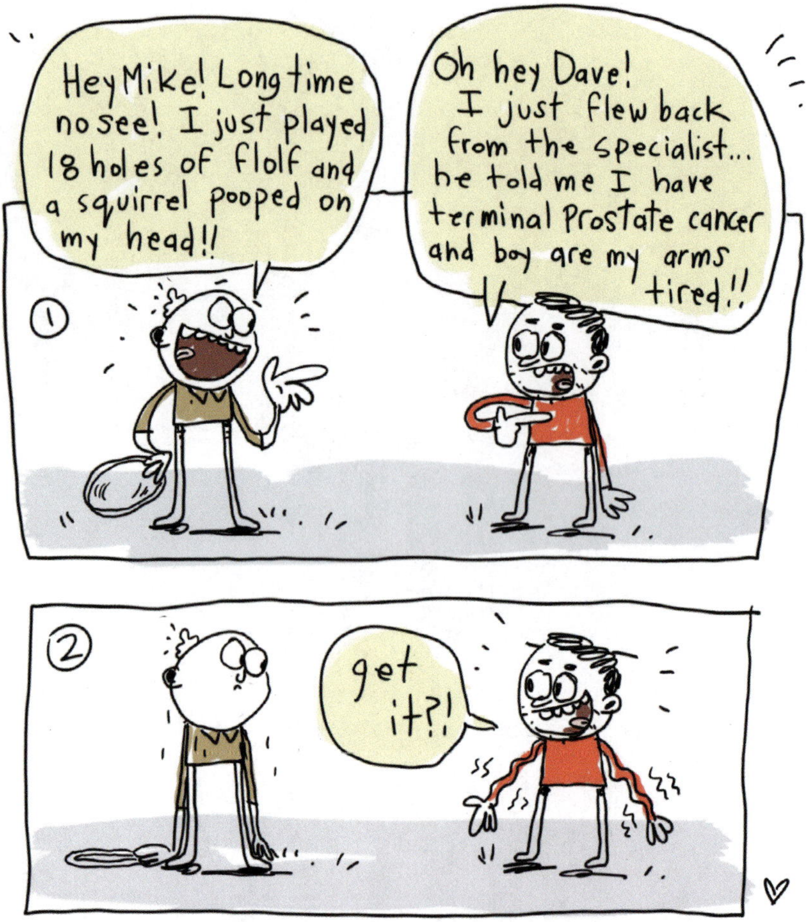
Hey Mike! Long time no see! I just played 18 holes of flolf and a squirrel pooped on my head!!
Oh hey Dave! I just flew back from the specialist... he told me I have terminal prostate cancer and boy are my arms tired!!
1
2
get it?!

Back Story: The Real Poop

Funerals and wakes are funny. The formality, the tension, the reverence, the ceremony, and the stories of the deceased can result in big laughs, especially when you're not the stiff.

But with a life-threatening disease, you're really playing to a tough room. While there is definitely tension, (spoiler alert) a cancer diagnosis also results in feelings of helplessness and futility, not the usual backbone for a good laugh, or even a real discussion. Nobody knows what to say or how to say it.

My family was raised with the Marx Brothers, *Blazing Saddles*, *M*A*S*H*, Monty Python, Richard Pryor, and most important, our dad, who taught us life lessons while busting a gut and showing the way past the bullshit to some hard truths.

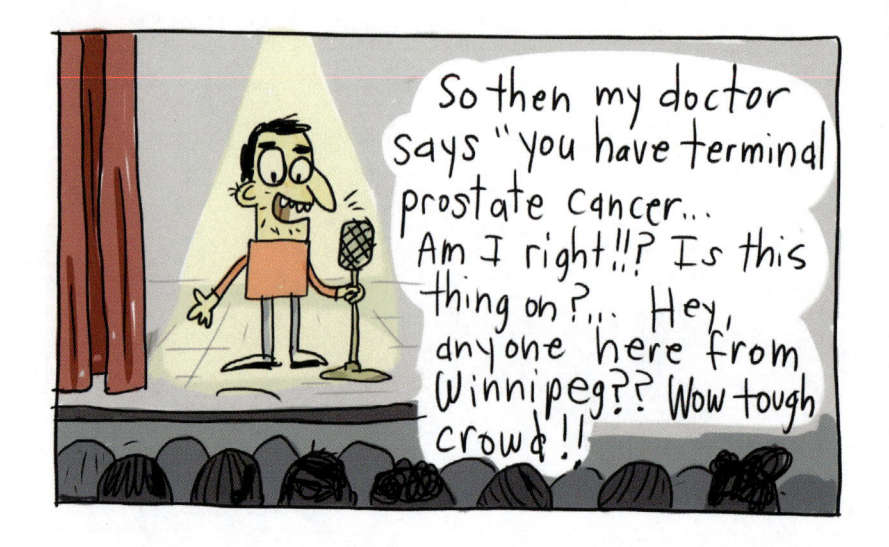

The last thing I want in my final years, months, and days are whispers and sad cow eyes from friends and family.

I've always been the type to whistle past the graveyard, so how can I do that now, before I take up permanent residency there?

By the age of forty-five, I had built a good life, with a wonderful wife and daughter, and a fifteen-minute walk from home to my own boutique consulting company, where I provided advice on the job market. I partied hard in my younger days but had finally settled down into a sweet routine. My favorite nights were no longer spent drinking until well past closing time. Suddenly, I was happy to have a good bullshit with friends, catch some ball, read a book, or watch TV in bed with my honey. I had a good thing going.

17

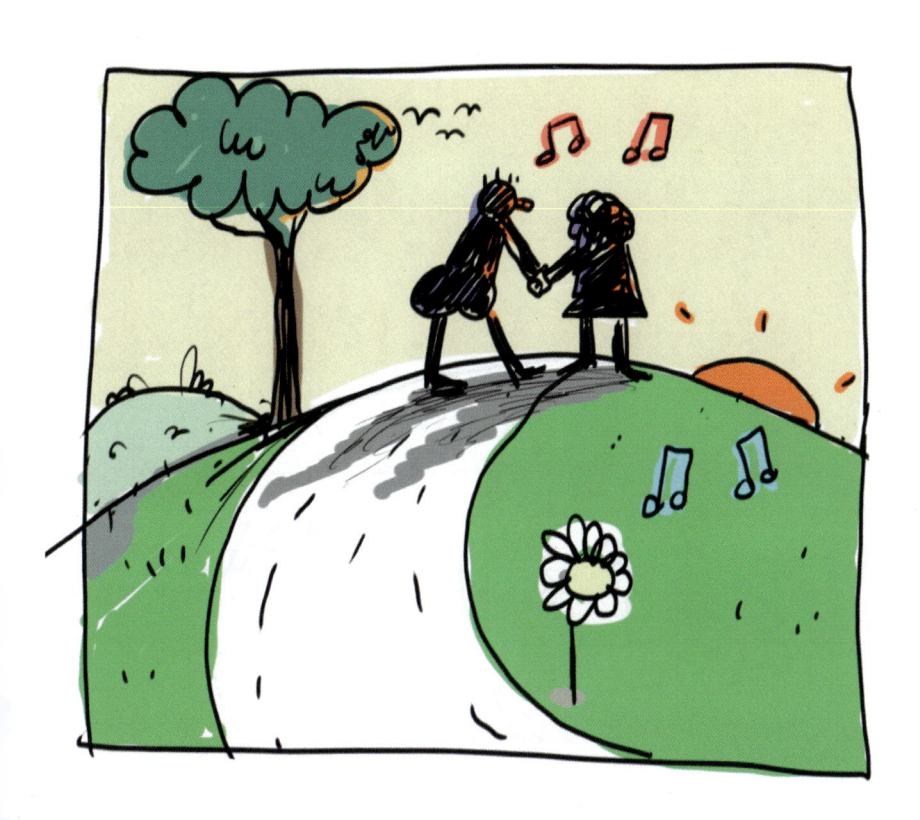

Michael's penis is kinda like his experience in the triple A basketball league... constantly called for double dribbling!

this penis joke is endorsed by chef BUDDY

Problem: Softwood Lumber Issues

When you're in your early forties, you never think it's cancer. Sure, some people do, I guess, but I didn't. I don't even think it is now.

More and more, I had to get up in the middle of the night to pee, but who doesn't? Or it took a few more shakes than usual to get rid of all the dribbles. No biggie.

After a while, I couldn't drive more than an hour in the morning without stopping at a restroom, but surely it was the big cup of coffee?

Then I had, as we say in mighty British Columbia, "softwood lumber issues." Now that's a problem. I was forty-two years old and I needed a little blue pill just to do what used to come quite naturally.

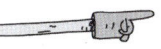

I was in good health, ate a good diet, and rarely got sick. Then, after a regular checkup, my family doctor sent me to specialists for the old finger up the bum. Several appointments went by, and all I got for passing my rump around the clinic like it was my first week in prison was "It's probably nothing. Try these antibiotics." Or, even better, "It might be in your head. Talk to the men's health nurse about your sexual relations with your partner."

I'm a guy. Talking about sex with a stranger is not something we do. Don't get me wrong, after a couple of drinks I'll brag about sex I had with *strangers* to just about anybody—except my wife. But most guys don't talk to other people about the real sexual relationships they have with their wives. It's in the vault. Besides, that wasn't the problem. There was a physical element that came and went.

And then it hurt. Not a lot, just a little from time to time, and a couple of Advil took it away. I mean, you don't cure cancer with ibuprofen, so it can't be cancer, right?

Besides, what does a sore prostate feel like anyway?

Well, now I know it feels like a sharp little turd you just can't pass and, believe me, I tried. I almost blew a major gasket on several occasions.

But, in this day and age, you have to be your own best health advocate, so I kept going back and insisting there was a problem. Not a big one, but I wanted it sorted out.

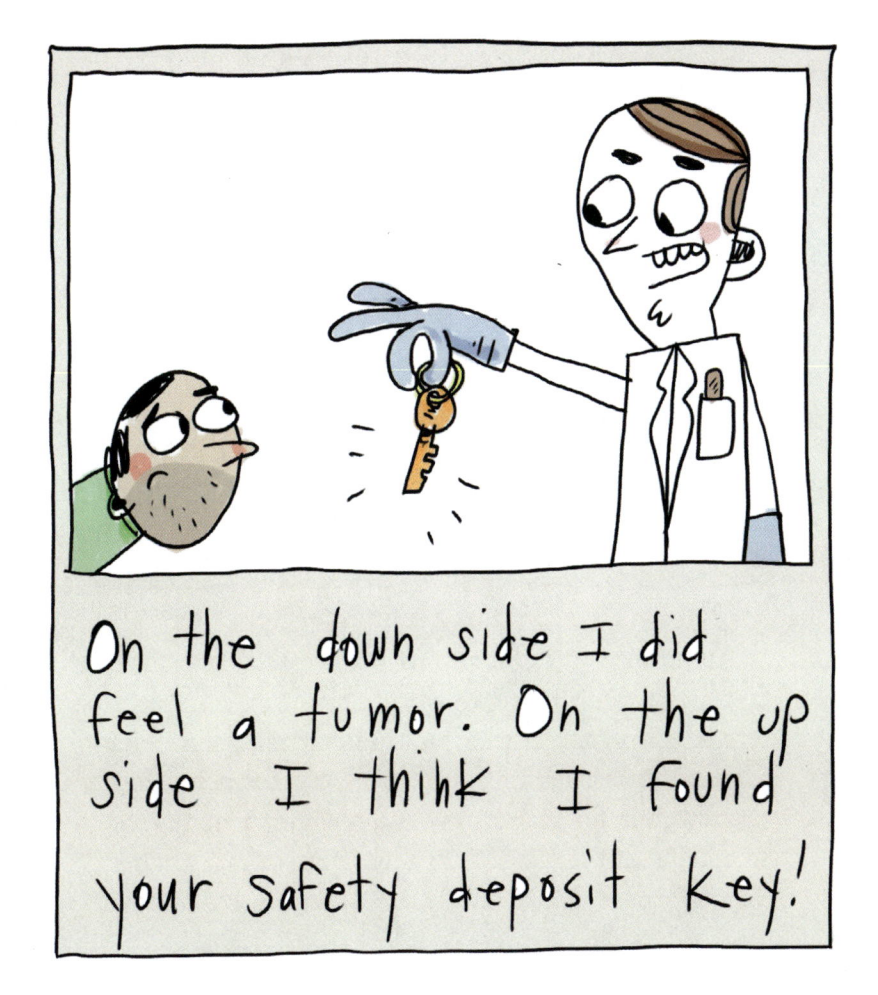

On the down side I did feel a tumor. On the up side I think I found your safety deposit key!

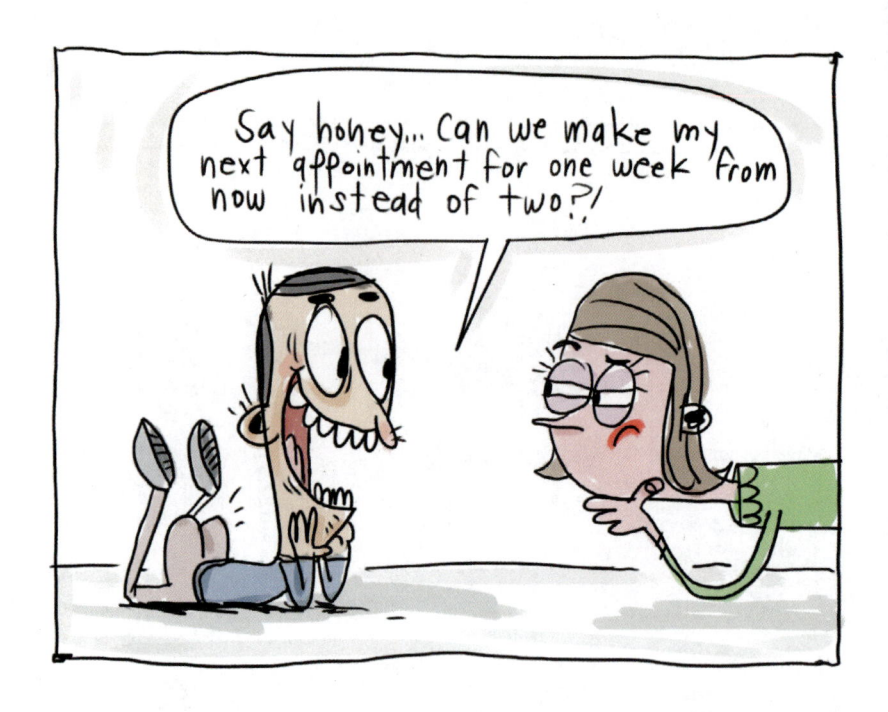

The finger up the bum test for prostate issues is a favorite of men around the world. In fact, avoiding prostate exams is one of the chief indirect killers of older men, as guys over fifty will miss appointment after appointment for years. And I don't blame them. It's not so much that the old digital exam hurts, but it is rather uncomfortable, and it really messes with a conventional sense of manhood.

Like most guys, I don't like dropping my drawers and opening my trunk for anyone, even my doctor, just to have them poke around in the exhaust pipe. Somehow, it doesn't seem right to have someone root around up there like they're looking for lost car keys.

At least it's over quickly and, most of the time, my doctor and I just clear our throats, look at the floor, and start talking hockey. After one appointment, I came back and told my wife that the entire exam was devoted to a full and frank discussion about which Swedes from the old Winnipeg Jets should be in the Hockey Hall of Fame. I was happy to report the doctor and I were in complete agreement about Anders Hedberg and Ulf Nilsson being underrated stars who got lost in the WHA amalgamation with the NHL. As for the condition of my prostate, we had no clue.

Now my wife comes to all my appointments. Now *that* is humiliating. The waiting room at the prostate clinic holds a bunch of old dudes with bowed heads, and our wives asking if we need to pee before the appointment.

So I say, "Stop being such a sissy! Lots of things are uncomfortable. Are you worried a finger up the bum is going to hurt, or that you're going to like it?"

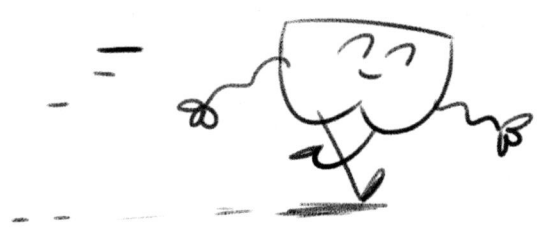

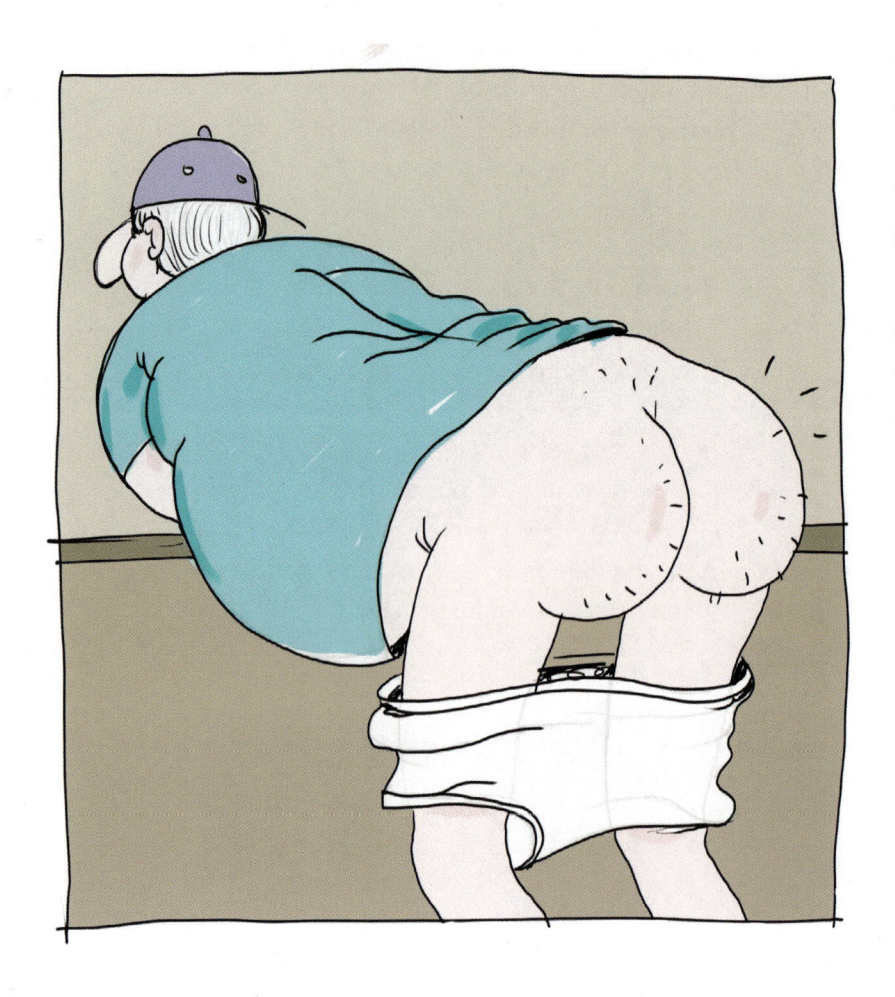

Tests: You're Putting That Where?!?!

F**ortunately, when looking** for prostate problems, there is a simple blood test for the prostate-specific antigen (PSA) levels, and in particular, for how fast this level grows, or doubles. For cancer, the PSA level is a marker, not an indicator, which means that you could have a rising PSA level that has nothing to do with cancer.

In my case, my PSA was increasing, but not too high and not too fast. So they sent me packing a few times. Nothing to worry about, because guys in their forties don't get prostate cancer, right?

They gave me some antibiotics to treat prostatitis, an infection of the prostate. It worked intermittently, which meant prostatitis wasn't the problem. The men's health nurse then suggested discussing sexual fantasies with my partner or role playing. My fantasy was for all this humiliation to end, and for everything to go back to normal.

However, since it wasn't prostatitis, it wasn't in my head, and guys in their forties don't get prostate cancer, the lead contender was something called benign prostatic hyperplasia, or BHP. As there is no direct test for BHP, and the treatment involves a cystoscopy, you want to be sure and rule out everything else first.

Let me be clear, you really, really want to rule out everything else first, because a cystoscopy is actually a tube they run up your penis to mess with your prostate. (Did you just wince reading this? I did writing it.)

I've never actually read Dante's *Inferno*, or seen the movie, for that matter, but I'm certain that a cystoscopy is the punishment in the ninth circle of hell, reserved for murderers, drunks who run red lights, and the inventor of user fees.

So, before that Roto-Rooter procedure, they sent me off for a biopsy.

Now, when you go for a prostate biopsy, they give you a choice between a general and local anesthetic. As a real man, I chose the local. Big mistake. When it comes to sticking long pokey sticks up the wazoo, I am now and forever a full-on wuss. "Knock me out, Doc!" If only I had known that then.

For some reason that probably has to do with legal liabilities or some other ass-covering procedure, the biopsy technician spent five minutes showing me these giant twelve-inch needles and grabby things, in order to explain how he was going to launch them up my back porch.

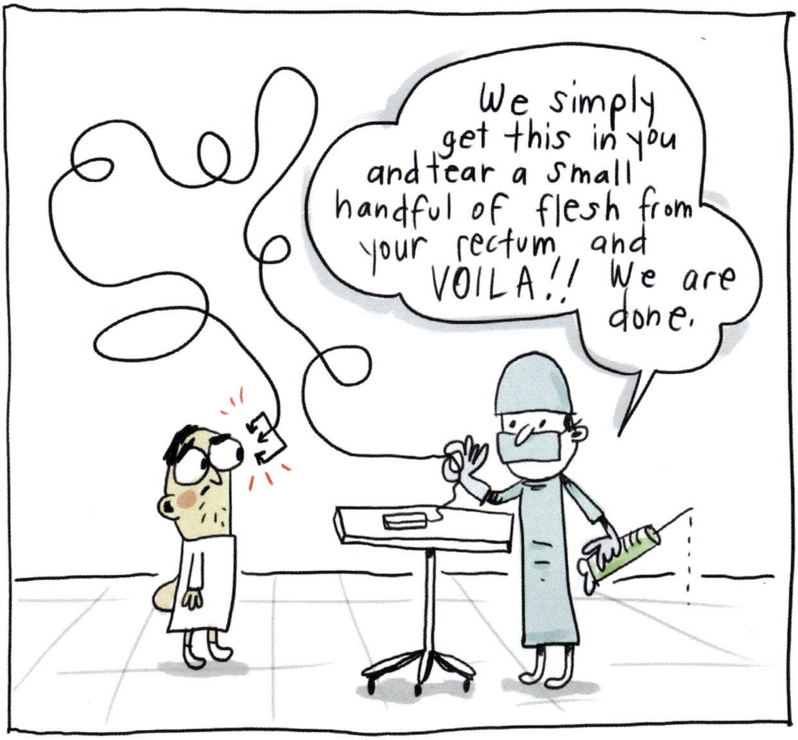
We simply get this in you and tear a small handful of flesh from your rectum and VOILA!! We are done.

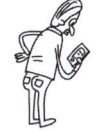

He was proudly telling me all this, and I was loudly yelling at him to stop showing me his arsenal. I didn't need the visual aids. I wanted to forget the whole damn thing, and it hadn't even started yet. Had I not been wearing the weird backless hospital dress, I may very well have bolted.

Eventually, we got down to it, or up to it, and he threaded the needle up my dark passage to freeze my rectum and my prostate. Somehow, enduring several pokes of a foot-long needle wasn't the end of the procedure; it was the beginning.

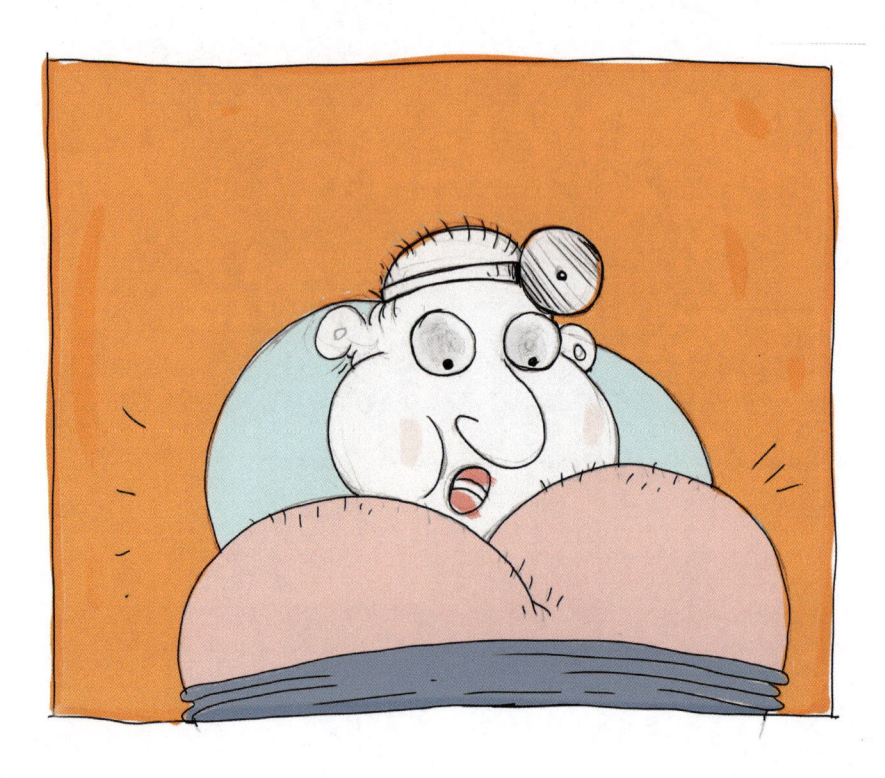

Once the freezing started to work, it was time for the other foot-long device. Mr. Grabby goes up the bum, pierces the wall of the rectum, pops into the prostate, and tears off a piece of the walnut-sized organ.

The first, second, and third times were just little tugs. By the fourth time, I could feel some yanking. I soon yearned for the days of old, of just having a finger doing the investigating.

But the fifth time took my breath away. It was... THE. WORST. PAIN. I've ever experienced in my life. It was like getting punched in the stomach and kicked in the crotch at the same time.

The technician asked if I wanted to stop and come back another day to finish the next five samples. "Are you kidding me? Five more!!!!" But no way I wanted to start over again.

When all ten samples were taken, I went home to painkillers and a twelve-hour deep sleep. Thank God that was behind me, so to speak. Soon, I would get the results and all this drama with the prostate would be over. I was a young, healthy guy, and dudes in their forties don't get prostate cancer, so nothing to worry about.

the stork

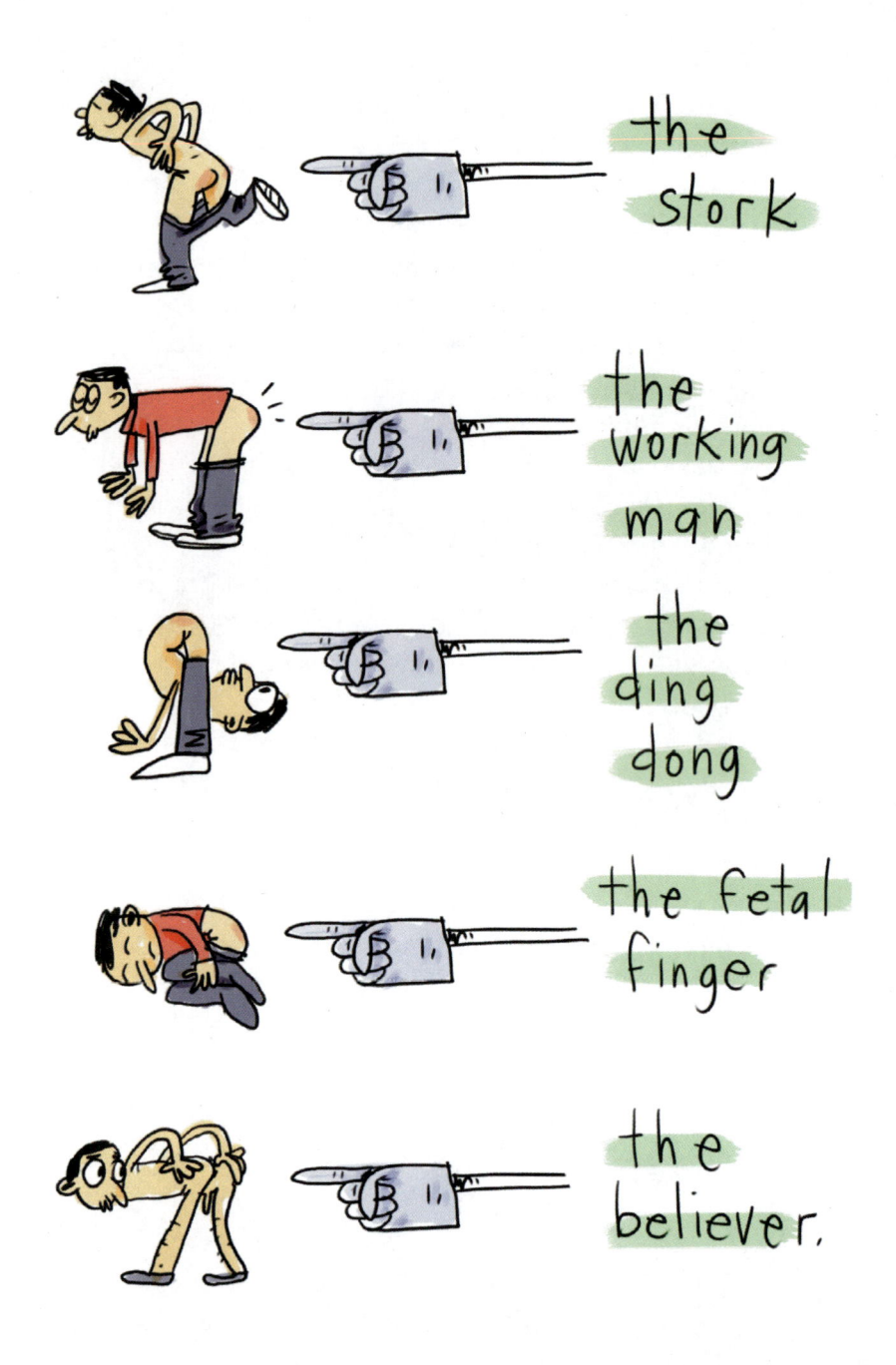

the working man

the ding dong

the fetal finger

the believer.

Diagnosis: Wait, What?

Along with the biopsy, there was also a bunch of specialists who wanted to cop a firsthand feel. From my family doctor to the urologist, to the proctologist, to the oncologist—they all wanted to put their finger directly on the problem.

As I eventually learned, each doctor has their own favorite method. Some have you stand and lean forwards onto a table, a most awkward and humiliating position. It really allows them to crank their mitts around in a 360-degree fashion, and allows men to experience some of the joys of childbirth. (Upon reading this, my wife laughed. "A finger up the bum is nothing compared to passing an eight-pound watermelon," she said. "Men are such wimps.")

Then there's lying in the fetal position, which is kind of my preference. Not because it hurts less—because it doesn't—but since I'm whimpering like a baby anyway, it's sort of the most appropriate posture.

Waiting for the test results of the biopsy, my wife joined me at the doctor's office, as she found my one-word reports of previous visits insufficient. In subsequent appointments this would become useful, as so often the doc would ask, "How you feeling?" and I'd say, "Pretty good." Then, as we both got up to leave, my wife would say, "What about the pain here, or the blood there?" And more often than not, pain and blood tend to be significant. Who knew?

But, in all fairness, the previous reports were brief because the medicos had no real answers, just speculation and possibilities. I have now learned that unclear answers are great, because definitive answers almost always suck.

Eventually, we got called from the big waiting room into the little waiting room, and after a few minutes of me playing with the plastic models of prostates and other weird things lying around, the doctor came in and said, "The biopsy took ten samples"—my legs crossed involuntarily—"and seven showed cancer with Gleason scores of nine out of ten. You have aggressive prostate cancer that should be treated immediately."

Well, that was pretty damn clear.

I was stunned.

My wife was stunned.

33

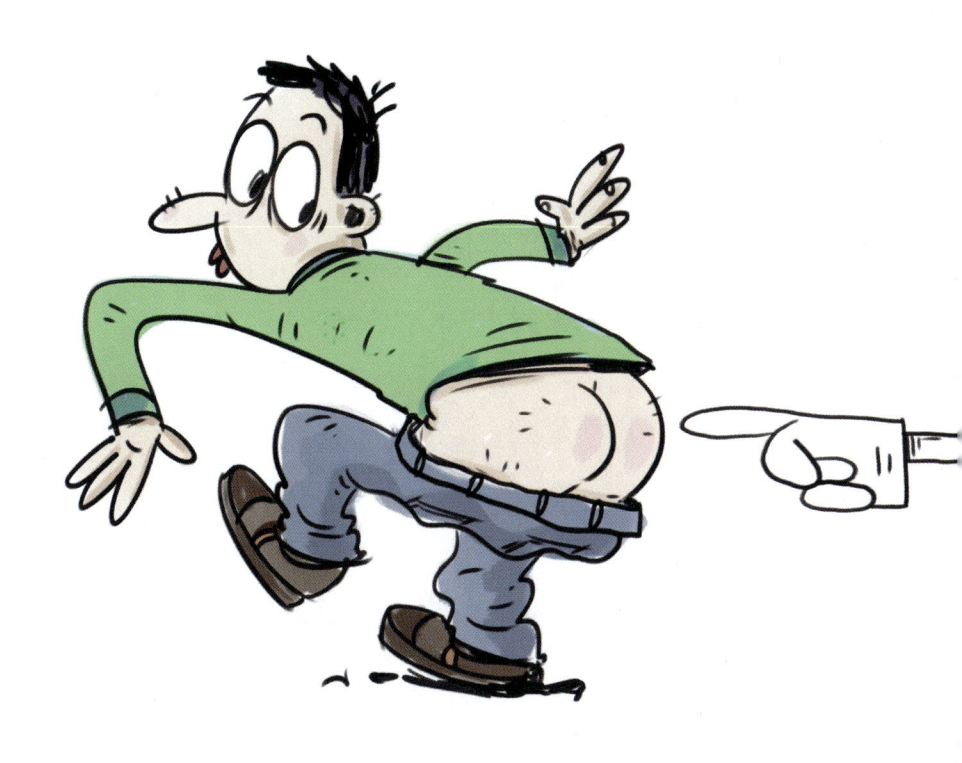

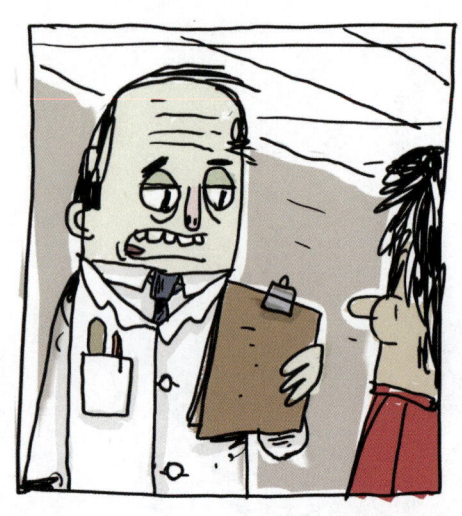

"People with your condition have a 60% survival rate in the next 5 years."

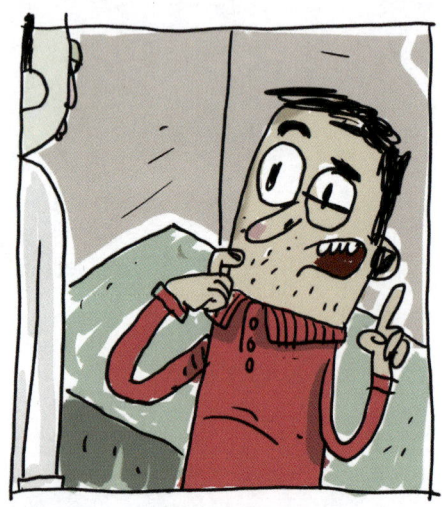

"Hmmm. I don't do math. Can you get me an abacus, someone that knows how to use an abacus and three extra strength pain killers..."

Other than having these few aches and issues, I thought I was healthy.

Apparently, guys in their forties *do* get prostate cancer.

He went on. "With the removal of the prostate and hormone therapy to follow, people in your condition have a 60 percent survival rate in the next five years."

I was forty-five years old. A 60 percent chance of making it to fifty! I was expecting better odds than that.

At every doctor's visit I've ever had, I have made at least one joke or comment that gets me the Look from my wife—you know the one I mean. But this time, we both stared straight ahead, and barely made a sound. Despite sitting next to each other, we couldn't look at each other, or even reach out and touch each other. We were both frozen, afraid that any human movement towards the other person would make this a reality, when, really, we both wanted this moment to disappear.

And then the doctor added a little uncertainty for old times' sake: "Unless the cancer has escaped the prostate capsule, and then we just don't know."

Wait, what?

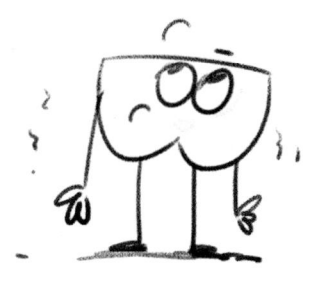

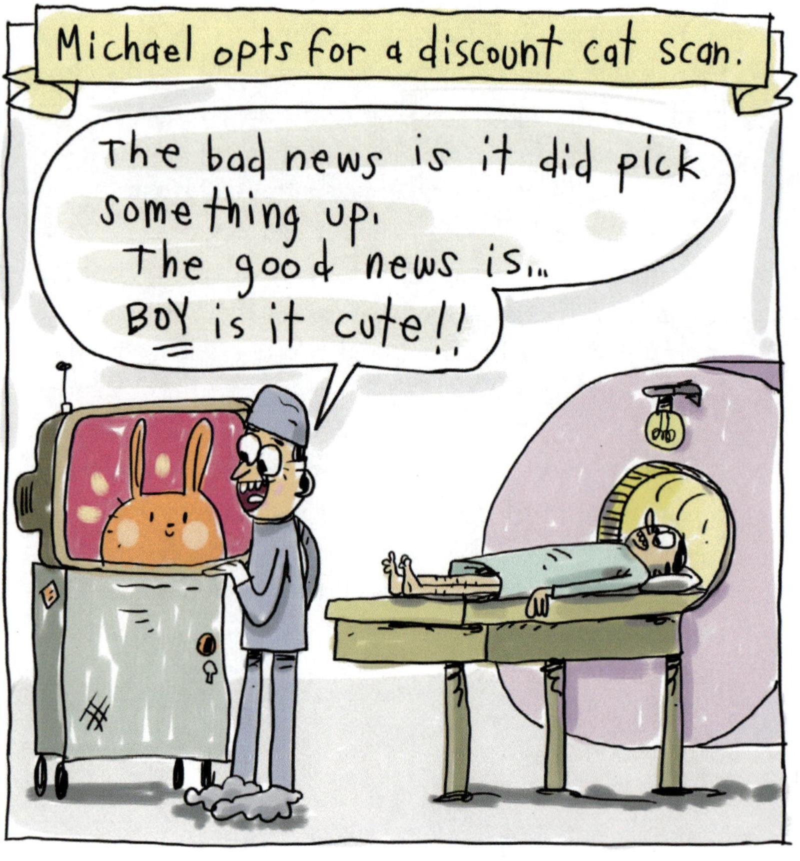
Michael opts for a discount cat scan.
The bad news is it did pick something up.
The good news is...
BOY is it cute!!

5

Surgery: I'm Still Using That

R**ight after my** diagnosis, they kept me busy with blood tests and the mighty machine tests, like a CT scan and a bone scan, to see if the cancer had spread to other parts of me. The CT scan is no big deal, as it's basically sliding through a big metal donut, but with no coffee.

However, the bone scan was a little freaky.

For the bone scan, they had me lie faceup on a slidey bed, which moved me into a big body-length contraption, with a hard, flat ceiling about a foot from my face. Then this ceiling slowly descended bit by bit, until it was a hair's breadth from my nose.

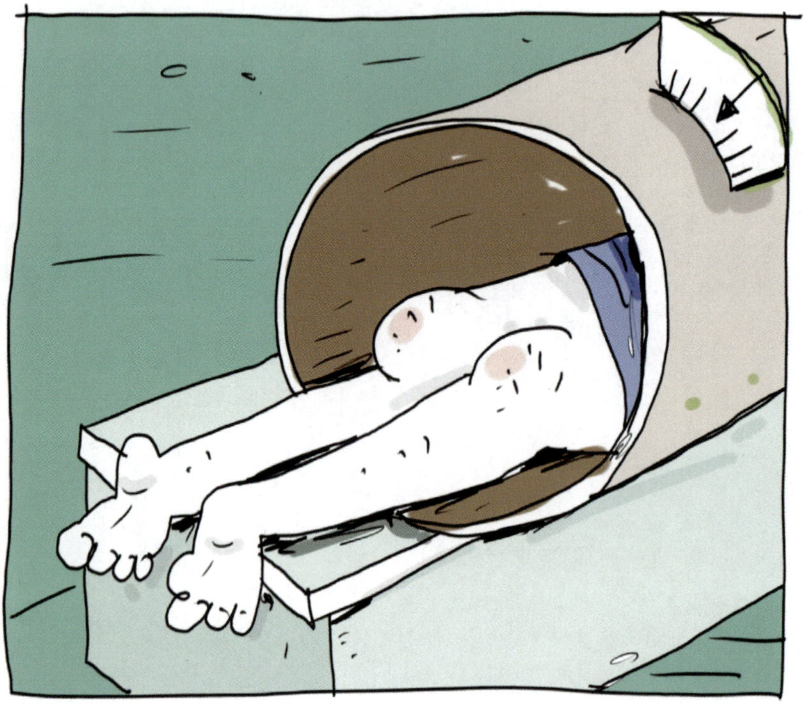

As it got closer and closer, I wondered when, or if, it would stop, because if it was even a split second too late, my nose would be crushed into my face. For a full twenty minutes, I stared at this metal ceiling, ready to scream if it made the slightest movement closer towards me.

Fortunately, the results all came back clean, and the cancer was not in my bones or any other part of my body. Unfortunately, I still have to get a couple of these bone scans a year, and every time it feels like sticking my head in a trash compactor and wondering if it will stop before it flattens my face.

Six weeks after my diagnosis, I had a radical prostatectomy. It sounds pretty cool, with the radical part and all, but that just means they took it out.

The day of my surgery, the two questions I was asked most frequently weren't "How are you feeling?" or "Can we get you anything?" No. Instead, for this crack medical team, from the hospital admissions clerk to the orderlies, the nurses, and the doctors, the question that seemed to be top of mind was "When is your birthday?"

Truth be told, I have absolutely no memory of the day I was born, despite the fact that it was clearly a very significant and traumatic day.

However, I guess they repeatedly asked for my birthday to make sure I was the right patient. I don't know why they don't go by names, but hey, it's not my hospital.

It was the second question that really concerned me. All the staff asked, "Do you know why you're here today?"

"Don't you????"

This didn't fill me with loads of confidence. Instead of continually writing down my birth date on the charts, couldn't someone jot down the type of surgery I was here to get?

Eventually, they checked me in, took my vitals, and loaded me up with Valium. It's a good thing they did, too, for, without the mellow yellows, I might have made a run for it, backless dress notwithstanding.

As they rolled me down the hallway into the surgical prep room with eight total strangers all strapping down different parts of me, they kept asking me over and over again, "Do you know why you're here today?"

In mere minutes, they were going to knock me out and do God knows what to me, and they didn't have this straight? It was bad enough they were taking my prostate and part of my manhood, but what if they removed something else, something that was working, and I was going to have to come back next week to do it all over again?

Or worse, were they planning to wake me up partway through to double-check?

Just as I thought I should make a break for it, the anesthesia hit, and I was out.

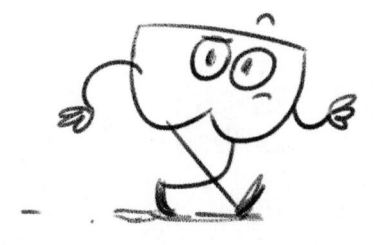

"Nurse, is this patient July 27? And if so, did he mumble he was in for a bum cheek lift?? It's always so hard to hear them when they are passing out! Ahhh... what evs!"

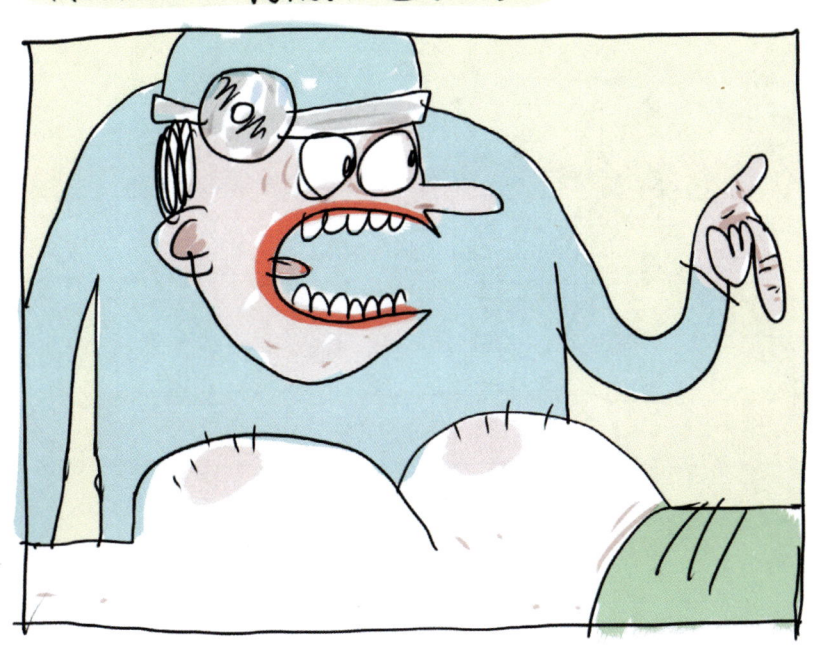

Michael seemed annoyed when he woke up from his surgery.

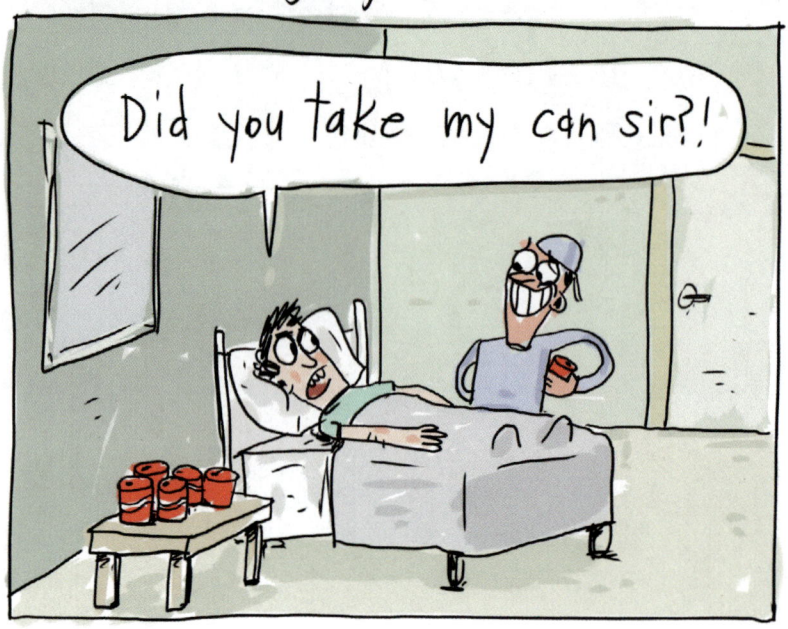

"Did you take my can sir?!"

Post-Surgery: What's That Coming out of My?????

woke up and realized I had survived.
This was a good sign.
My eyes opened and I saw the most beautiful sight I had ever seen. My wife looked like an angel. I don't know if I was just so happy or just so very stoned, but I fell in love all over again.

Good thing, too. I was in a daze yet woke up saying all the right things to the woman who was about to nurse me back to health. Who knows what I could have said under the influence. What if I said another woman's name? What if I was a surly prick? What if I accidentally gave out my PIN? These are powerful drugs and should not be used lightly. They should really warn a dude about this.

My second thought was that I had to pee. I asked the nurse for a bedpan or something, and she smiled and walked away. I asked my wife for help. She rolled her eyes and pointed at my bedside.

When they removed my prostate, they also took other good stuff like nerves, muscles, and part of my urethra. So when I awoke, there was a catheter in place—a plastic tube coming out of a place no man wants to see a tube. The catheter ran all the way from my bladder through what was left of my tallywacker to the outside world and into a bag hanging beside my bed.

This may have been necessary, but it was also truly horrifying. It was like a bad episode of *Star Trek*—My Penis of Borg.

Then, after one night in the hospital, they sent me home with loads of pills and extra pee bags. The pills weren't as good as the ones in the hospital, but not too shabby. The problem was that they blocked any bowel action, so I had to take more pills just to keep the trains running.

Now, imagine me sitting on the loo, trying to make things move along for number two, while my body is battling medications, and I've got a tube coming out of my Johnson to take care of number one. The logistics were complicated, to say the least, yet they were an essential part of every single day.

The first day, I lowered myself gently onto my home throne and gave the usual squeeze to get things moving. But this little thrust also pinched muscles that scooched my catheter about a half inch through my willy.

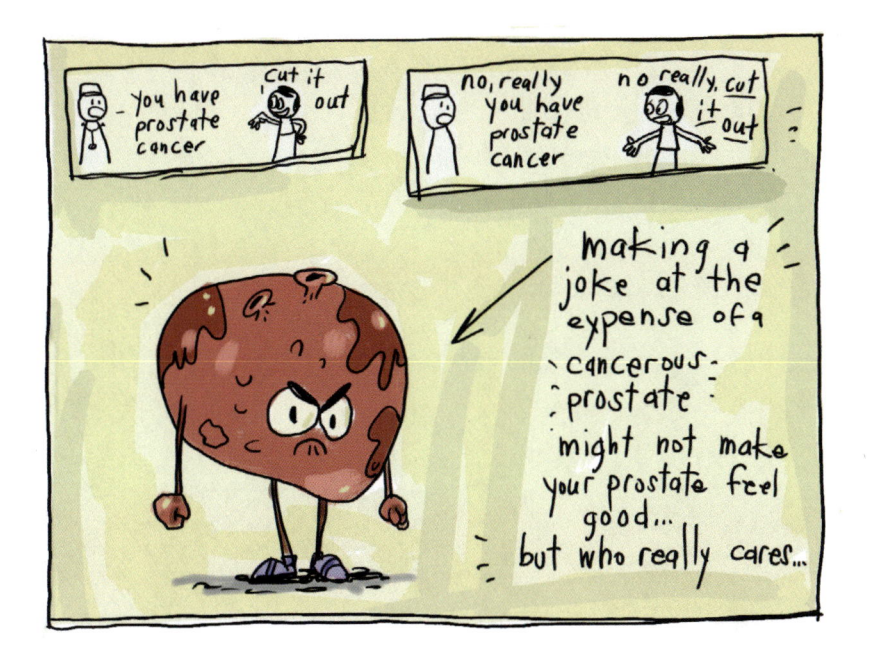

In truth, my high-pitched scream was more surprise than actual pain, but it brought my wife rushing to the bathroom, and had the neighbors wondering if they should call the cops. I think it even set off a few car alarms.

Needless to say, on the second day, I took a much more conservative approach, yet managed a little action anyway. Since friends and family were always looking for an update, I was only too happy to oblige with all the details of my BMs they could handle. Soon enough, they stopped asking.

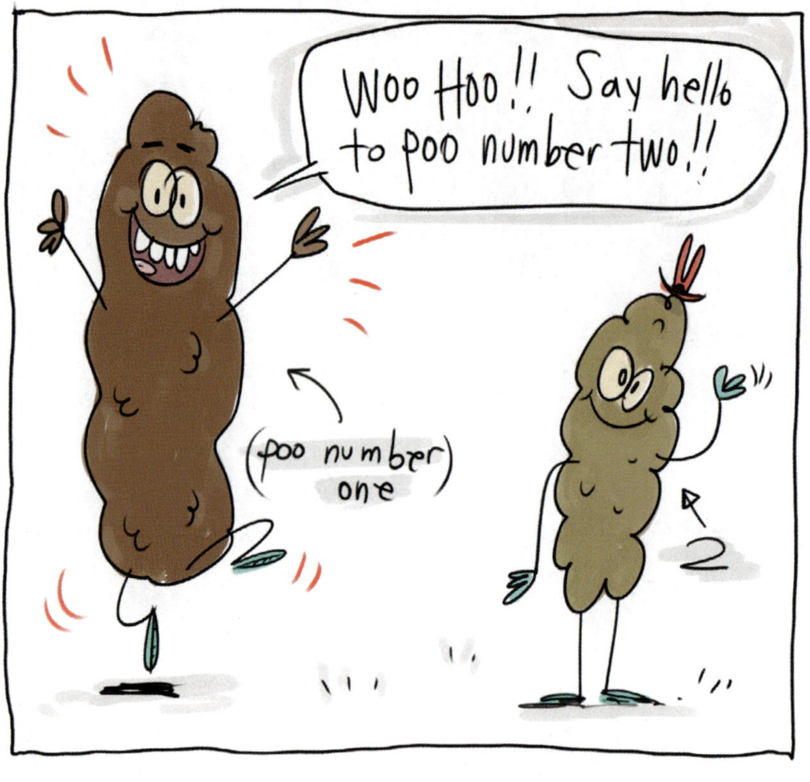
Woo Hoo!! Say hello to poo number two!!
(poo number one)
2

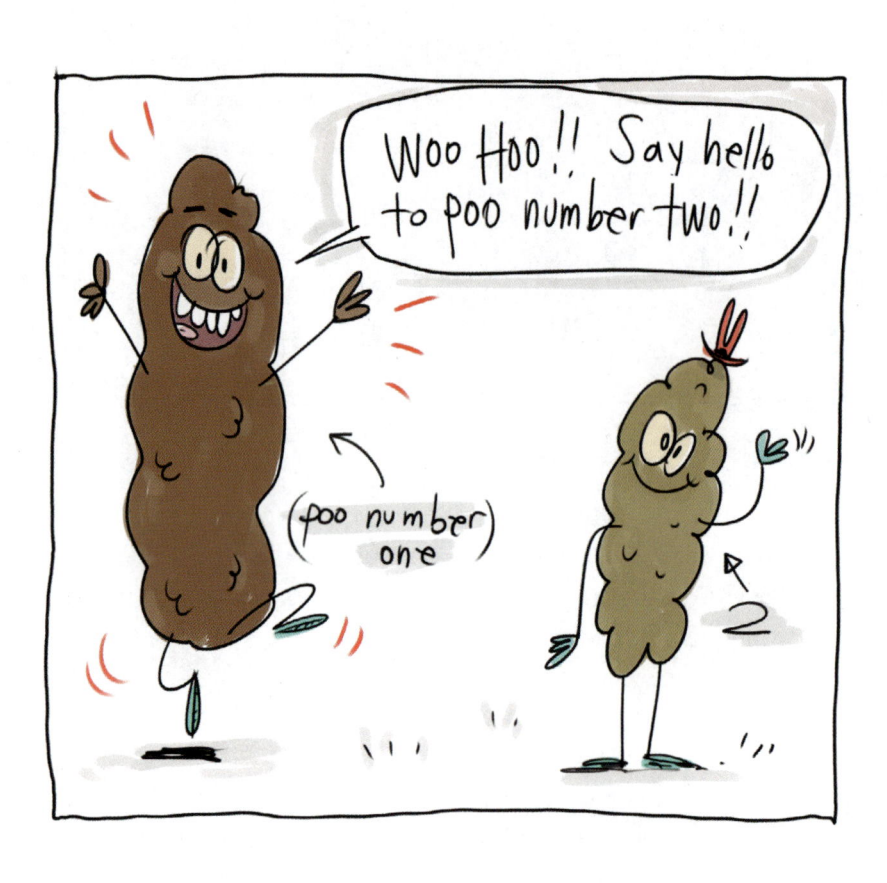

The first week after surgery was intense; it was all about the little things in life. Taking a shower was a miracle, walking around the living room was cause for celebration, and regaining control of my bodily functions was a top priority. After one week, I visited my doctor, who removed my catheter with one long yoink, and a most surprising *pop*. These damn treatments were almost worse than the damn cancer.

The thing is, without the prostate and some of those muscles and nerves, I had to teach my bladder to hold my pee, something I hadn't had to learn since I was three... or five... Who am I kidding, right, Ma?

It wasn't easy and it wasn't fast. A rubber mattress cover, pee pads, and even diapers became part of my routine, while I gradually built more control through Kegel exercises, and lots and lots of squeezing. At first, I had very little control; in fact, the flow would start as soon as I sat up or changed position. So anytime I sat down to eat, or watch TV or whatever, I had to have everything I needed within reach, because whenever I stood, I had to make a beeline for the bathroom.

Even now, after I have regained control, a good cough, sneeze, or laugh, and all bets are off. My wife says, "Welcome to my world."

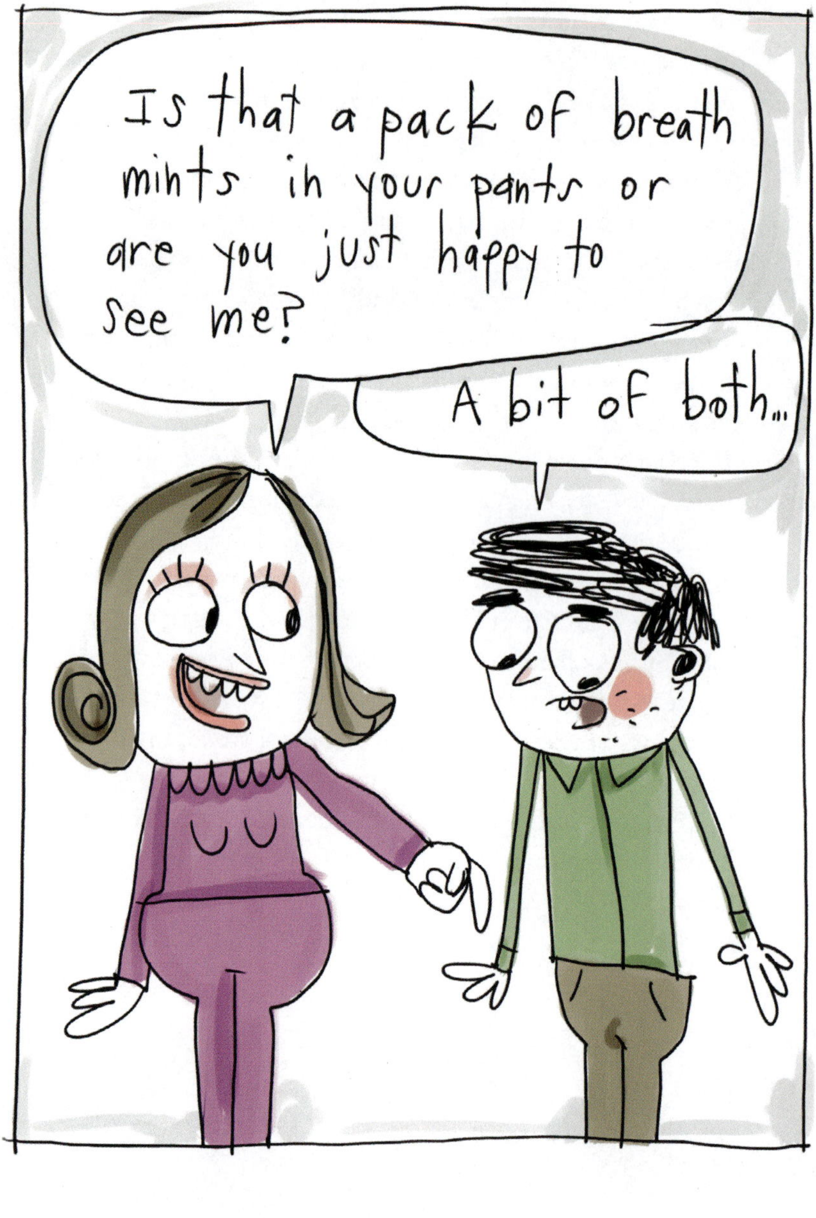
Is that a pack of breath mints in your pants or are you just happy to see me?
A bit of both...

Hormones: Chemical Castration—That Doesn't Sound Good

Whew! Did it get hot in here all of the sudden, or is it just me?

Women deal with fluctuations in hormones all the time. Men may also experience those fluctuations, but we just don't know it, or perhaps just don't recognize it. We most often put it down to hunger.

One of the most common treatments for prostate cancer is hormone deprivation therapy, as the hormone testosterone acts as prostate cancer food. The idea is to cut off the food source to starve the cancer.

Soon after my surgery, I took a daily anti-androgen pill for a year, and four times a year a large capsule was injected into my belly fat for a slow dissolve.

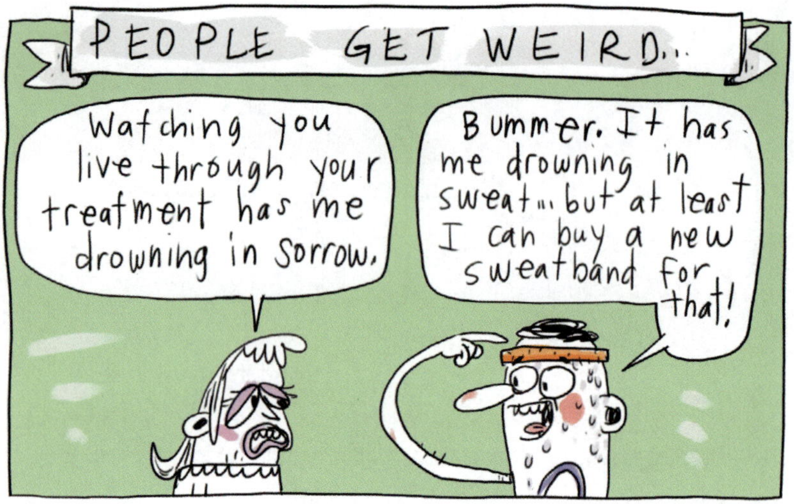
PEOPLE GET WEIRD...
Watching you live through your treatment has me drowning in sorrow.
Bummer. It has me drowning in sweat... but at least I can buy a new sweatband for that!

Finally, I was well prepared for one of my treatments, as I had built up a nice padded deck over the years and it gave the capsule a sweet home. Together, the pills and capsules worked to block the production of testosterone in my body.

For well over a year I had hot flashes—like ten to fifteen times a day I broke into a full-body sweat lasting about five minutes. I'd be in a movie, or a meeting, or even in bed, and I'd rip off every piece of clothing that was socially acceptable—and a few that weren't.

You could even see me jump out of my car at a red light, peel off my jacket, sweater, or T-shirt, and jump back in, just as the light changed. Once the hot flash passed, naturally I was cold and had to put everything back on.

Other than fatigue, a big appetite, and a few headaches, the side effects were pretty good. I still had a great mess of curly black hair on my head, but the hair on my arms, legs, chest, and back disappeared—kind of a win-win, really.

There was just one problem, and a pretty big one at that.

Sex.

Or rather, what's that again?

You see, when you cut off the testosterone in this manner, it is also known as chemical castration. But no matter how you cut it, that's just not good.

Since I was a young, randy lad, the right look, touch, thought, or glance led to a physical chain reaction in my brain and body that was all natural and fully integrated. I know now, those messages were sent through hormones.

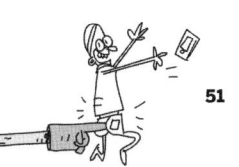

While the first sexual thought, glance, or touch still gets my attention, the reaction kind of just stops there. In days gone by, I would think of baseball to slow things down; now I must stop thinking of baseball just to keep things going.

As for the softwood lumber issues? Well, when you remove the prostate, the nerves, and the testosterone... forget about it. That ship has sailed. I still have the sensation of touch but not the same connection and sense of anticipation. Sure, pills, pumps, and straps can help, but it's often a lot of sound and fury signifying nothing.

I have even tried a concoction that I inject directly into my fallen warrior. I sat in the bathroom with a shaky hand holding a needle, trying to line up the right spot in between veins and arteries, at the correct angle and depth. This was just about the worst aphrodisiac I have yet to come across. Some dudes may be into that kind of thing—pay for it, even—but not me. Call me old-fashioned, but I prefer not sticking sharp needles into my little guy.

But you can't keep a good man down for long. Thanks entirely to a beautiful, sexy, skilled, and extraordinarily patient wife, my finish, while having no flourish, is stronger than ever. When you move sex from the body to the mind, I've found that it can be more intense than I ever thought possible.

SO MANY QUESTIONS...

Is it possible that my prostate developed cancer out of anger stemming from wearing a bladder hat its entire life?

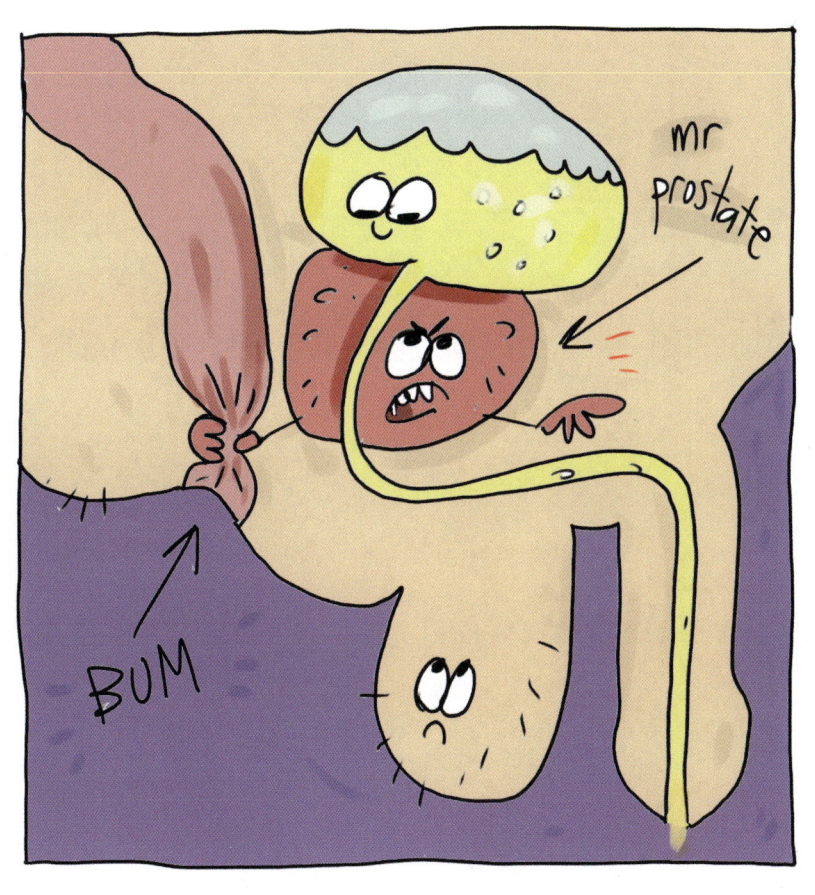

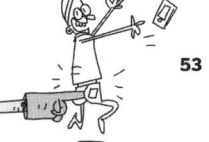

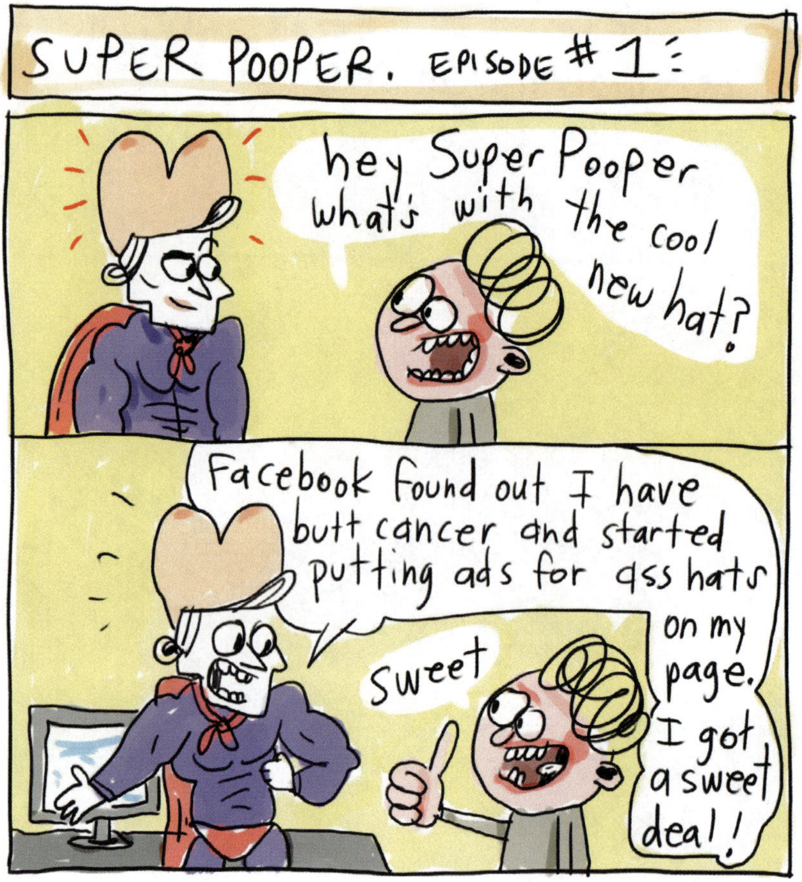
SUPER POOPER. EPISODE #1:
hey Super Pooper what's with the cool new hat?
Facebook found out I have butt cancer and started putting ads for ass hats on my page. I got a sweet deal!
sweet

Radiation: The Origins of a Superhero!

"**We want to** try radiation to shrink your tumor. Do you have any questions?"

Cool, I thought. *Both superheroes and supervillains are often created through doses of radiation.*

"Do I bring an insect or some other creature for me to absorb its traits, or does the hospital supply one?" I asked.

It didn't really matter what I said, though; by this point in the proceedings, the doctors had stopped talking to me and only addressed my wife. Over two years' worth of appointments, the doctors had eventually realized who came prepared to talk medicine, and who came just to make smart-assed remarks. Yet they continued to address her anyway.

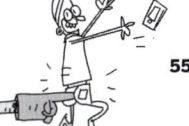

My wife asked, "What are the side effects of the treatments, and what's the prognosis afterwards?"

I mean, I guess those are good questions, too.

Three years after my surgery, and a year after the course of hormone treatments ended, I felt pretty good. My PSA numbers were low and were growing slowly. I ate a healthy diet, dropped thirty pounds at the gym, and was in the best shape of my life. Even the once-lifeless love muscle started to come around and show some interest again.

Except for one thing.

After a while, I started to spend more and more time in the bathroom. My guts moved things along, but the back passage was a little blocked at the exit.

Then the bombshell.

My quarterly PSA results, which had risen from 1.8 to 2.4 to 3.2, jumped all the way to 24!

The cancer was back with a brand-new tumor in my bladder and rectum. When prostate cancer spreads, it usually goes to the bones, specifically the big bones like the back and hips. Not for me. While the docs repeatedly sent me for those near-face-crushing bone scans, my cancer secretly made a nice home in soft tissue. The funny thing was, when it moved other places, it was still called prostate cancer, even though I no longer had a prostate, because the cancer cells were actually prostate cells.

Since prostate cancer feeds on testosterone, the doctors put me back on hormone deprivation therapy. Hello, old friends—hot flashes, big belly, and shriveled up... well, you know. But in three months, my PSA scores went down from twenty-four to five.

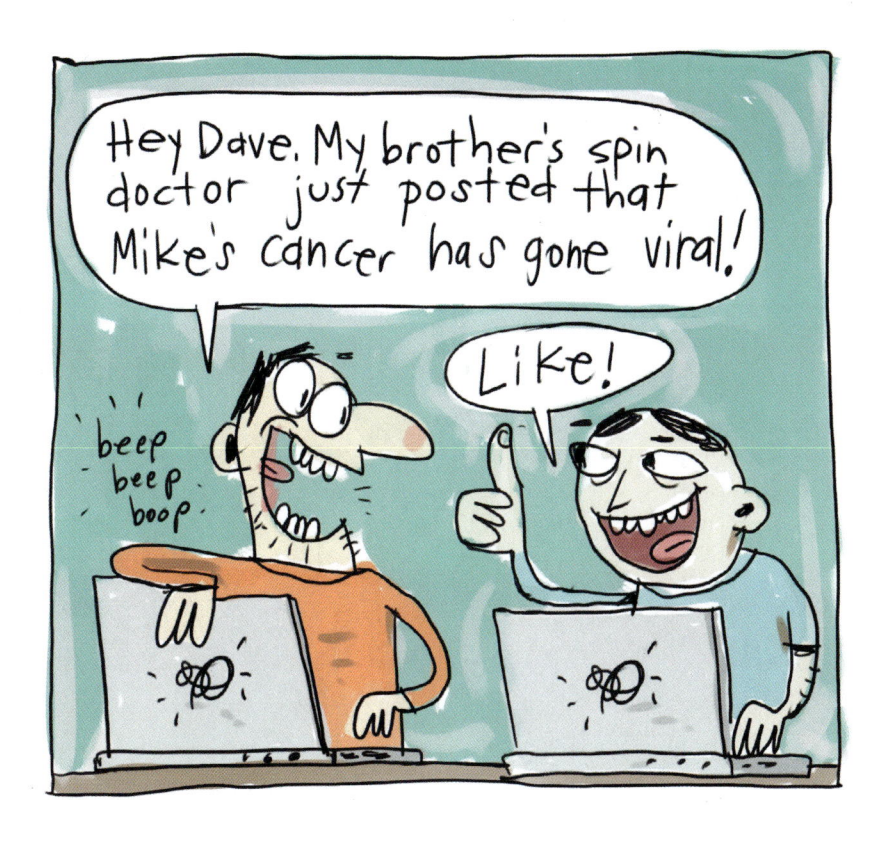

They also scheduled me for radiation to target the tumor where the sun don't shine. Radiation for me was twenty-eight five-minute X-ray-type procedures, conducted five days a week for about six weeks. Pretty easy; I didn't feel a thing.

They even gave me three tattoos, little dots on my hips and belly to line up the radiation perfectly each and every time. They look like homemade tats of punctuation marks. Not so much badass prison ink—more like tramp stamps from grammar camp.

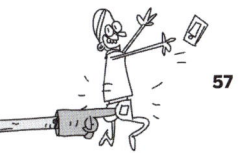

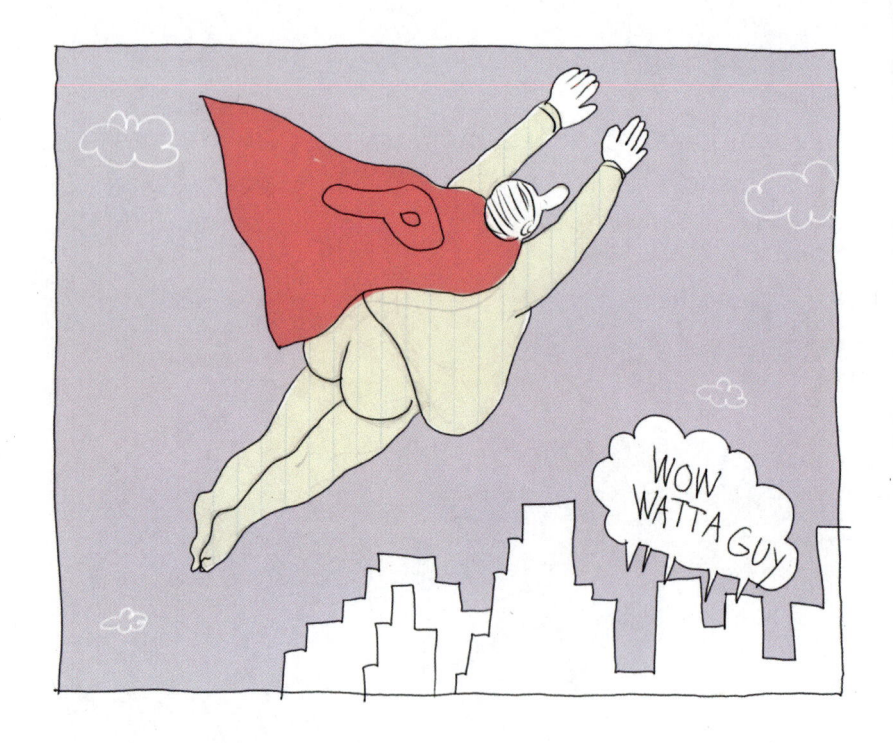

Since they were blasting my strike zone, they wanted me to come in with a full bladder to protect some of the healthy bits inside. The problem was they were targeting that area because I had problems holding number one and letting go of number two. So I drank lots of water on faulty tubing with no relief for an hour—ensuring that five minutes of the procedure were an exercise in Zen-like concentration. As soon as the blast of radiation was over, I did a super-fast small-step shuffle to the bathroom, and came uncomfortably close to another nautical disaster.

Side effects of radiation are usually cumulative, which means things start off slow and build over a couple of weeks. Not for me. Almost immediately, I had aches and pains, and my old problems with blocked bowels soon became a tsunami in the other direction, which isn't too surprising considering the Hiroshima treatment they were giving my rectum.

Codeine and other pills helped but left me cloudy and not really alive. So, after years of prodding from friends, I tried something I had given up thirteen years earlier, but this time it came in capsule form—cannabis oil.

Once this liquid chronic hit, my symptoms were relieved in one sweet wave. Now instead of feeling cloudy and dead, I felt happy and alive, ready to go back on tour with the Stones. The stress of the radiation was gone; it was like a reset button.

How is this stuff not standard issue?

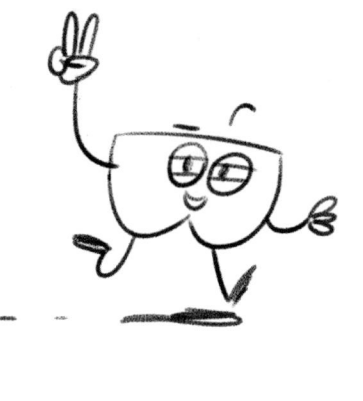

*If you are a travel agent, please use your best judgment when advising cancer of its possibilities for vacation locations... thx.

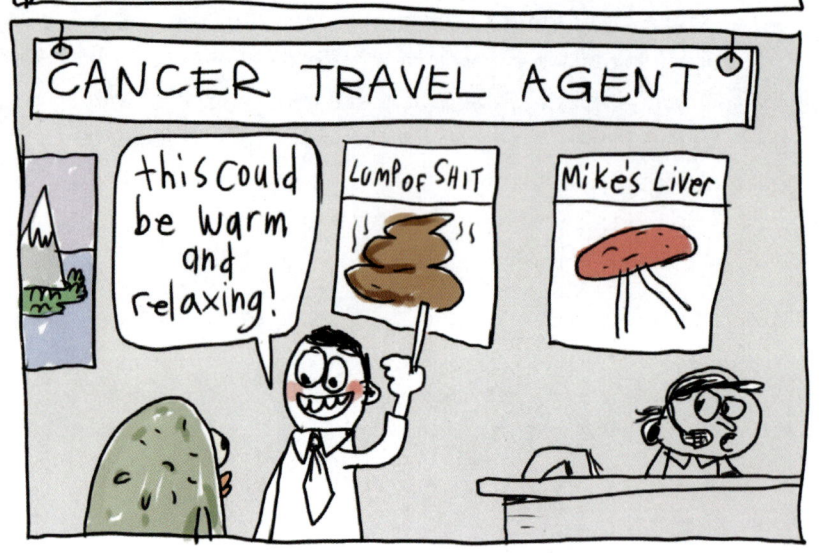

CANCER TRAVEL AGENT

this could be warm and relaxing!

LUMP OF SHIT

Mike's Liver

9

It's Still Not Working: Trials and Tribulations

The problem with aggressive strains of cancer is that they don't follow the usual patterns and don't always respond to the usual treatments.

My hormone deprivation meds worked for six months into the second course of treatment, but then the cancer started to adapt. The radiation may have shrunk one tumor, but it couldn't stop the spread. It also didn't result in any superpowers *whatsoever*. Good or evil, I would have been happy either way.

The cancer spread through my blood, which is bad in itself. This meant it was no longer a local thing with surgical options. Not that I was looking forward to my doctors coming after me piece by piece. "First we take your bladder, then we take Berlin."

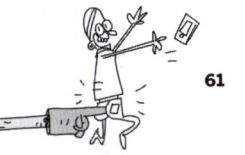

The inmates had escaped and were running wild. For now, they are hiding out in my liver. I recently checked Wikipedia and apparently you need your liver to live. I think that might be how it got its name. But, hey, I'm not a real doctor.

Usually, I have to ask my doctors to give me an estimate of how long I have left. I get anywhere from a few years to a few decades. Well, I could have guessed that. It's hard to plan out your life with all of these maybes.

My three doctors are like the three bears. Doctor #1 (Baby Doc) tells me, "Well, if everything works out, you could live another thirty years." Doctor #2 (Mama Doc) just hums and haws: "Let's wait and see. It really depends on a lot of things."

But once the cancer had spread to my liver, Doctor #3 (Papa Doc) asked me if I wanted to know my prognosis. Not a good sign.

I thought I was prepared for the answer, and I knew it wasn't going to be good. I thought I had maybe three to five years left. After all, I was in great health... except for the cancer. But, even then, the answer was a shock.

"On average, people in your condition last about one year."

Thud. Only one more birthday, one more anniversary, one more round of play-offs, one more Christmakah. On the bright side, only one more tax season and no more trips to the dentist.

If my four year old son would give my brother advice on what to say to a doctor after he gives you some very heavy news...

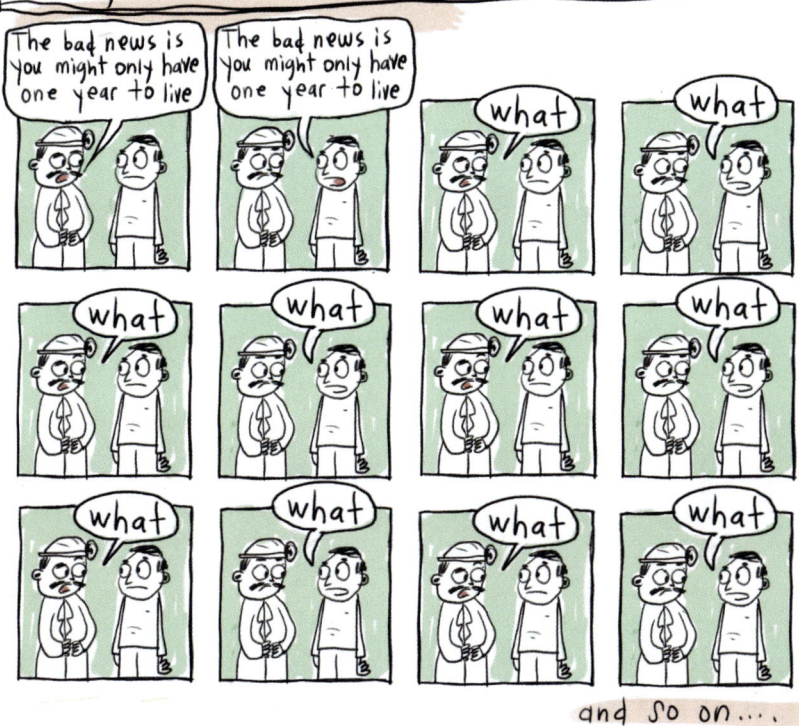

The bad news is you might only have one year to live	The bad news is you might only have one year to live	what	what
what	what	what	what
what	what	what	what

and so on....

More good news for Michael

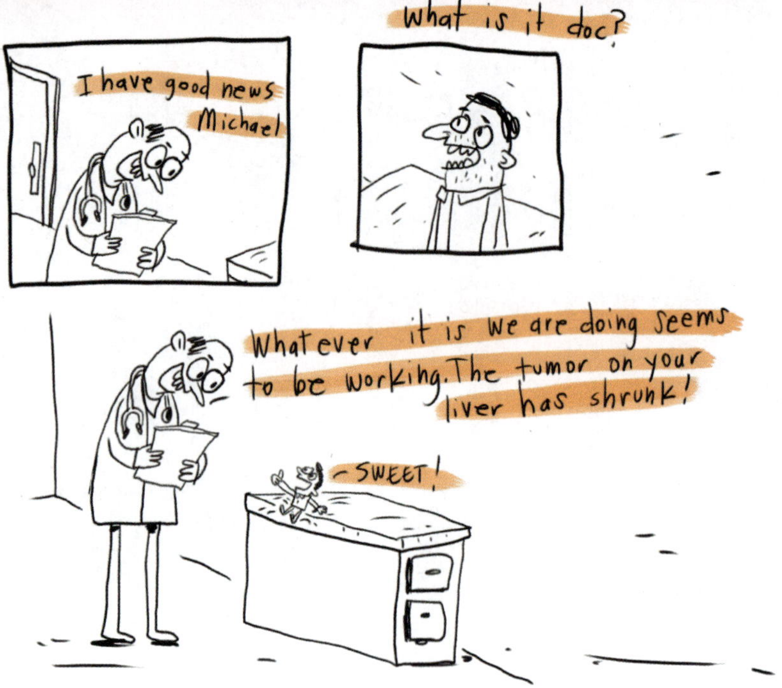

For most people the so-called bucket list is an expression; for me it was a giant ticking clock in my head.

Sure, there is always hope for some new medication or another, but the cancer is in my liver, so the best they can do is delay the inevitable. There is no cure. At least I am not yet at the stage where they are offering to make me comfortable.

So now I've signed up for a few clinical trials, and luckily the first of the new meds seems to be working. Hopefully, this buys me some more time, because I'm not ready to go.

It's not so much the bucket list of things to do. A trip here or fantasy camp there, a Vegas blowout or writing the great novel isn't at the top of my list anyway (though, technically speaking, I did just write this book). Quite frankly, a bucket list is what you make up when you have all the time in the world. Besides, I did that shit in my prime; I don't need a greatest regrets tour. In any case, between the side effects of the meds and getting older in general, my energy level just ain't what it used to be.

I'm not looking for more time to rewrite my life; I only want more of what I already have.

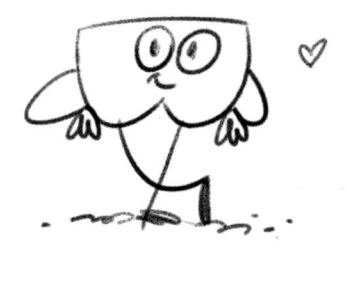

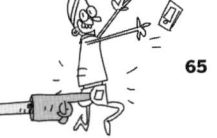

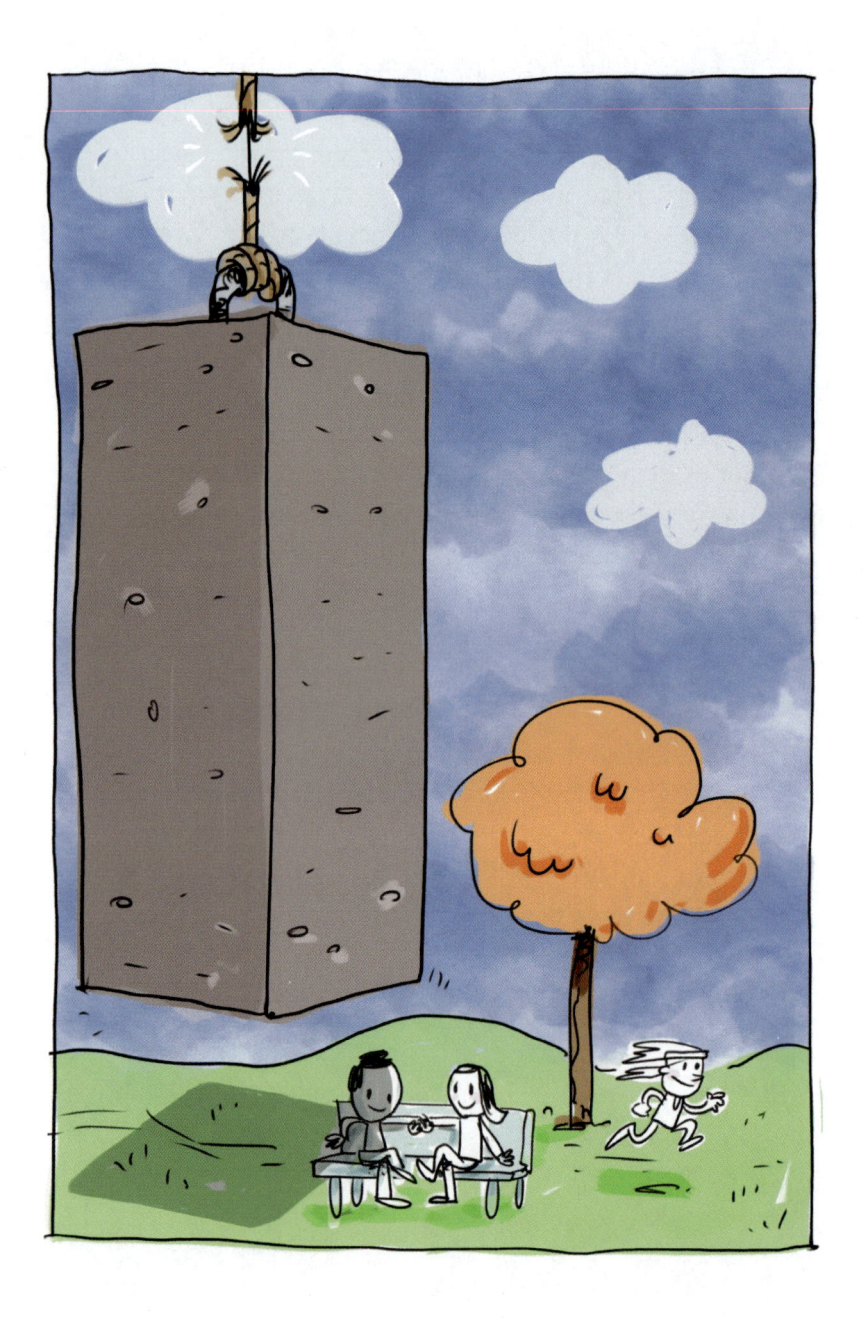

10

Hang on, I'm Not Dead Yet: The Meaning of Life, and Other Great Movies

A **few months have** gone by in my new time-limited reality, and life has returned to pretty much normal... whatever that means.
Bills to pay, work to do.
Que sera, sera.
Sunrise, sunset.
Chop wood, carry water.
Ob-La-Di, Ob-La-Da.
Life is life.
No future but what we make.
Get 'er done.
Carpe diem.
YOLO.
Pick any cliché that fits your culture or mood.

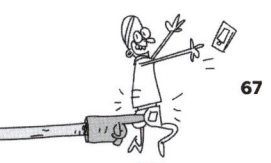

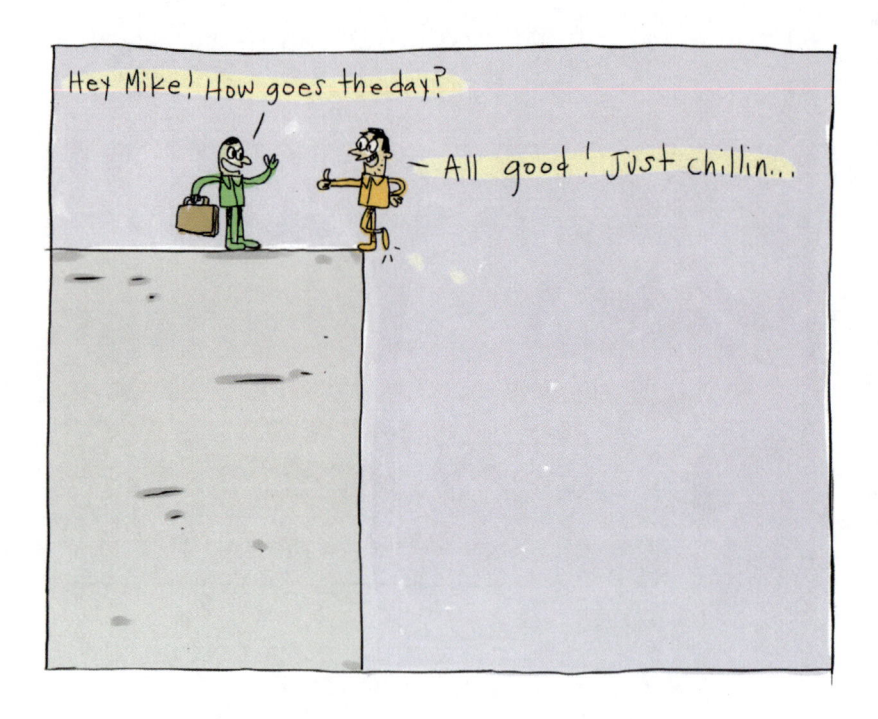

The truth is that when you're living with dread what you want—or what I want, anyway—is to be normal: a normal day, a normal life. I want people to treat me normal, and I want to feel normal.

Because when it comes right down to it, we just don't know when our time is up. Quite frankly, we all come with an expiration date. Sure, I have a window into a possible exit, but I could just as easily get hit by a bus.

In fact, eight years ago, my youngest brother, Jon, was cruising down the highway to make a meeting about a cartoon emergency—apparently, they have these quite a lot. Out of the blue, a fully loaded semi trailer T-boned him and his car spun out of control. The car was crushed, and Jon was lights out. Amazingly, he woke up in the hospital, with aches and bruises but essentially all right.

Our dad has been living on borrowed time since he had a five-month stay in several hospitals in 1981 with pancreatitis. Since then, he's had diabetes, a triple bypass, delirium from time to time, weird things with his feet and toenails, and now Parkinson's—along with bad eyes, bad knees, constant colds, and multiple falls to break a few ribs for good measure. Two months before my prostate surgery, he went under the knife to get a bacterial infection of unknown origin scraped out of his shoulder... for realz. The old man is damn lucky just to be an old man. No wonder he's so damn grumpy.

None of us really knows when we're getting called up to play in that great big gig in the sky. So I plan to enjoy myself. Spend time with my friends and family, listen to some old rock 'n' roll, watch some good TV in bed with my lovely lady. I will keep working because I like my job, and I need the money. And you can always find me at aquafit at my local pool because I still have to stay in shape, and get the latest neighborhood gossip.

All with one thought in the back of my mind.

Today is a good day to die... or maybe next Tuesday.

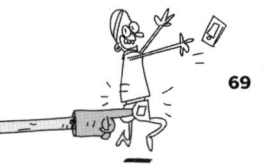

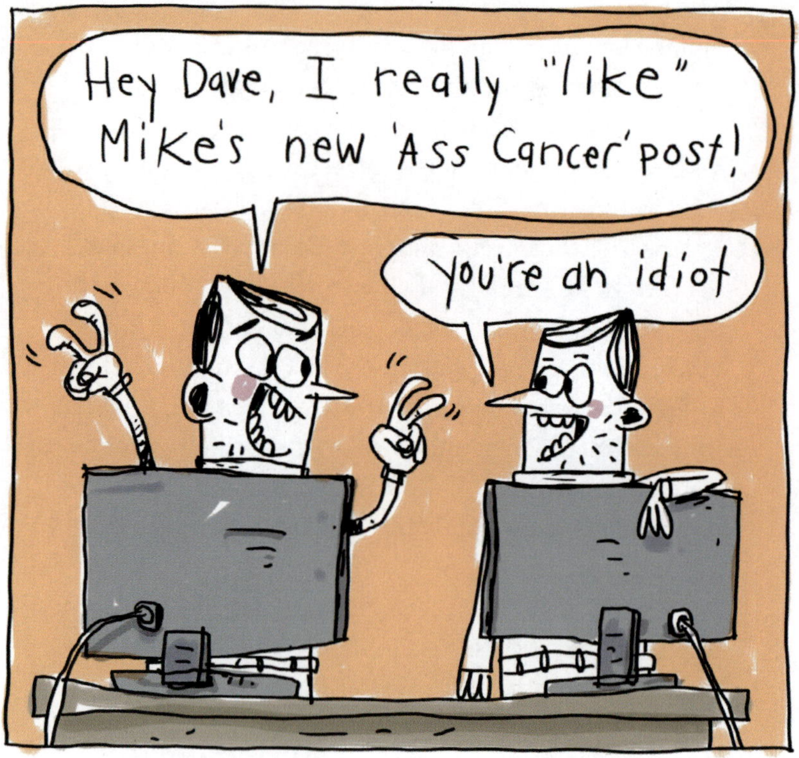
Hey Dave, I really "like" Mike's new 'Ass Cancer' post!
you're an idiot

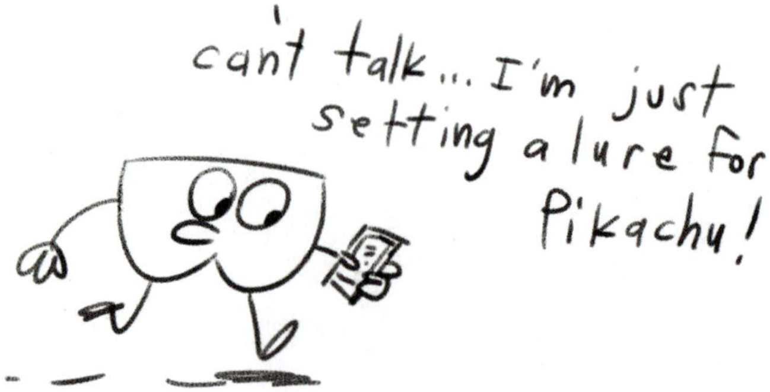
can't talk... I'm just setting a lure for Pikachu!

Rear End Notes: A Family Affair

When I was first diagnosed with prostate cancer, my wife, Gina, created a Facebook page to keep people updated. It had one rule: tasteless comments only. "Not Fans of Mike's Ass Cancer" helped keep people informed and me smiling. While I'm sure our posts and comments might have offended some people, they can all get stuffed.

And no one was more tasteless than my brother Jon.

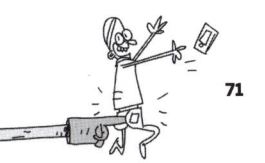

Like our dad, my youngest brother is a great artist. By day, Jon is a director of animated TV series like Cartoon Network's *Supernoobs*, Teletoon's *Dr. Dimensionpants*, and Network Ten's *Dex Hamilton: Alien Entomologist*. Gina and I even wrote a couple of episodes of Jon's very own series on da CBC: *The Very Good Adventures of Yam Roll in Happy Kingdom*. We wrote the good ones.

By night, Jon came up with a few cartoons to help him get through my cancer and make me laugh. Sure enough, between my stories and his cartoons, we made others more comfortable—or uncomfortable—with having a real conversation about my cancer. So with advice and encouragement from Gina, we decided to make a book. (This very book, actually.)

Then a funny thing happened. Jon sprained his wrist making a diving catch between the head of his teetering toddler and the corner of a coffee table. The kid was all right, but Jon's drawing hand was buggered. With a delay in developing illustrations for this book, our dad, a retired architect and a grumpy but funny old bugger with his own mad skills, asked if he could add a few cartoons. Great!

As the head of the family, my dad has often felt helpless in this cancer business, and it was an unfortunate barrier in our relationship, as we lost the ability to communicate with each other. But as soon as he was able to draw things out—his medium—things changed, and we're now able to have healthier discussions about my illness and life in general.

So, with a life-threatening prognosis hung on me, we thought we'd take a stab at sharing our stories and drawings with others.

Besides, it's not like I'm an eight-year-old with eye cancer or something horrific like that. I've got prostate cancer, and it may be terminal, but it also means stories about pee, poo, and (no) boners—basically, the trifecta of humor for twelve-year-old boys. And I haven't met one guy yet who has really, truly evolved beyond that. My wife agrees.

While I wish we didn't have the reason to make this book, I'm glad we got the chance to share it.

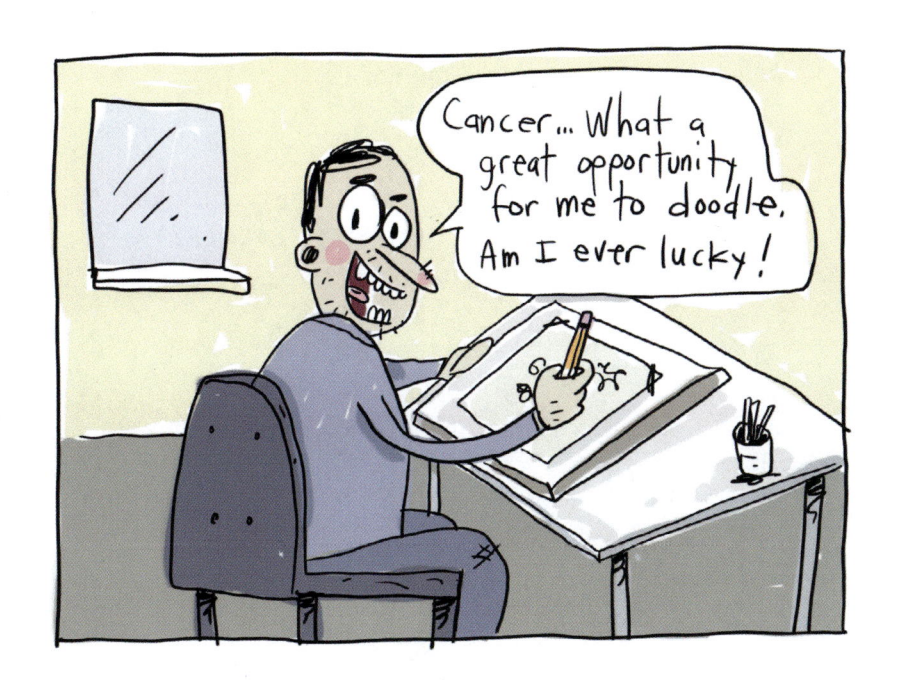

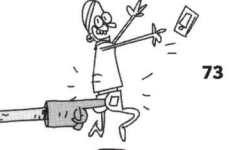

Finger Fighters

Far too many people are struggling with cancer and other diseases. Thank you to those who provided support for this book, and we want to recognize those close to you who know the struggle. You are not alone.

Russell Barnlund
Bob Benner
James Clark
William Harry Coreau

Susan Darrell
Stormin' Norman Duncan
Art & Pearl Edmonds
Robert Kenneth Fidler
Elvira Fiorino
Nurit Fox

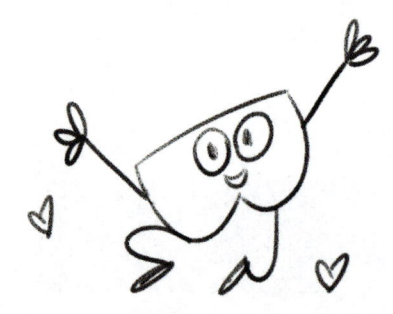

Don Graham
Lindy Greenberg
Luigi Guercio Sr.
Jerry Guitar
Chuck Herman
Kanako Kariya
William & Mary Kuzyk
Val Leclerc
Kee Ban Lee
Nancy Lieth
Alan Charles Mar
Shelagh McInnes
Chief Roy Mussell,
    Sxela':wtxw till

Austia Palmer
Myrna Roy
Varya Rubin
Stephen Savauge
Bill Southworth
Dino Taronno
Dale Underwood
Graham Walker
Willem White
Jerry Woolsey
Chris Wootten
William Paul Zubyk

you made
me blush,
thanks!

Wall of Fame

The *Finger up the Bum* team thanks and recognizes the contributions of our big donors, who really helped make this book possible.

Marta Demong
Justin Dyer
Barbara Izen
Peter Killam
Sherry Krawitz
Rick Kuzyk
Ashley Ramsay
Alex Rueben

Lovey Sidhu
Val Madrien Smith
Queenie Tse
Wazuku Advisory Group
Deb Young
Brad Zubyk

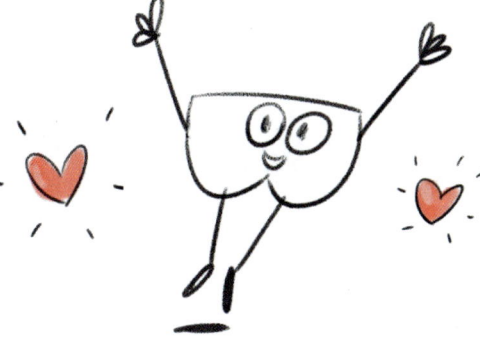

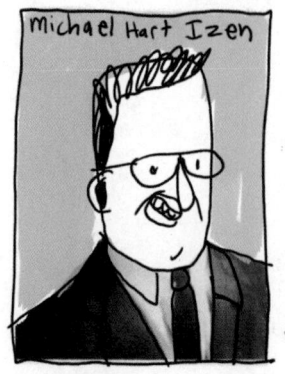

michael Hart Izen — "want a book?" ← nice suit

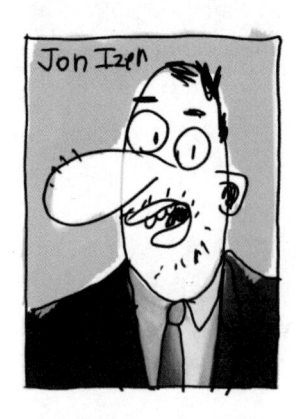

Jon Izen — "want a banana?" ← borrowed suit

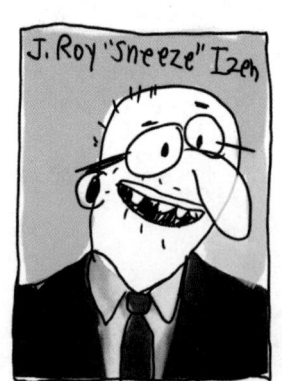

J. Roy "Sneeze" Izen — "want a half a banana?" ← discount suit

About the Creators

Michael Hart Izen · Cancer Boy: At forty-five years old, Michael had a happy life with his wife and family, and was running a boutique consulting firm, when he was diagnosed with aggressive prostate cancer. At forty-nine, he wrote this story with family and friends.

Jon Izen · Brother of Cancer Boy: He made these corking cartoons to deal with his own anxieties about Michael's cancer and to make his brother laugh.

J. Roy "Sneeze" Izen · The Old Man: As the father to the Izen boys, he instilled a strict discipline of cartoons, jokes, and irreverence.

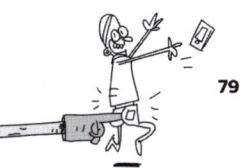